D0472205

SHOP
YOUR
CLOSET

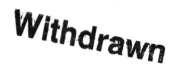

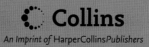

An Imprint of HarperCollins*Publishers*

SHOP YOUR CLOSET

The Ultimate Guide
to Organizing
Your Closet
with Style

Melanie Charlton Fascitelli
with Kevin Clark

This book is dedicated to my father John C. Charlton, Jr., the person who made me ambitious and instilled the confidence in me that I could be anything I wanted to be.

HarperCollins books may be purchased for educational, business, or sales promotional use. For information, please write: Special Markets Department, HarperCollins Publishers, 10 East 53rd Street, New York, NY 10022.

FIRST EDITION

Designed by Lorie Pagnozzi and Reshma Chattaram
Illustrations by Keith Geldof
Photographs by Douglas Friedman

Library of Congress Cataloging-in-Publication Data has been applied for.
ISBN 978-0-06-134381-0
08 09 10 11 12   ID3/IM   10 9 8 7 6 5 4 3 2 1

CONTENTS

SECTION TWO
IN THE CLOSET

SECTION THREE
STAYING ORGANIZED

Chapter 9: From Closet to Suitcase   119

The ins and outs of packing, and how your closet plays a pivotal role

Chapter 10: What to Do When He (or She) Moves In   129

How to make room for your significant other and their wardrobe

Chapter 11: Beyond the Closet   137

Other areas of your home can benefit from the principles applied to your closet, from your medicine chest to your pantry, from your bookcase to your CD/video collection

FOREWORD

When I began my company a few years ago, I learned an important lesson: Nothing good comes easy. *Shop Your Closet* is an actualization of that lesson. After several rewrites of the initial proposal, switching coauthors, meeting with literary agents, and almost bagging the entire project, we finally arrived at this point—a book articulating my vision. This book represents the brand, the design niche, the lifestyle mantra that my company, Clos-ette, is today.

The best thing about the Clos-ette vision is that it was an underdog; no one really thought it would take off. And many didn't see the niche market I was trying to create. I heard time and again, "I don't get it." Luckily, *Vogue*, which wrote the first editorial piece on us, got it, encouraging me to stay focused and on vision. Slowly, I became better at explaining our mission, and people began to understand the value and the need for organization in their busy lives. Today, Clos-ette is a holistic organizational design firm, a cabinetry business supporting organizational design ideas and ideals with a comprehensive accessories line to further enhance and achieve the organized lifestyle we all strive for.

Did it matter if anyone thought that a company based on a little girl's obsession with clothes, closets, and organization would become a comprehensive business, complete with actual employees, offices, and individual retirement accounts? Not really. I believed in Clos-ette from day one; I knew that a lot of people liked to "shop their closet," so I figured out ways to make it easier and more fun. I felt that it was my personal goal (actually, my duty) to clear the clutter in people's closets (what I like to call their clogged wardrobe chi) and instill a sense of serenity within their master walk-in by putting things in order and awakening the hidden Buddha buried beneath the piles of clothes and layers of stuff.

Shop Your Closet is part how-to workbook, part design guide, and part style notebook. It is a written manual of how we approach our work at Clos-ette and how we accomplish the goals needed to enhance our clients' lives. Our secrets and insider tips to styling, organizing, designing, and building closet spaces are clearly and concisely contained within this book to help you begin your journey on the path of organization and clutter-free closets.

Shop Your Closet has been a path of self-discovery. It allows me to share with you all the things that I have learned from building Clos-ette: the joy of working with wonderful clients in their beautiful homes and enhancing their lives by creating beautiful closets and organizing their chaotic spaces into serene havens. It also is a culmination of my years in my former career putting together retail spaces and stores, while editing and styling my own wardrobe and personal spaces. But the greatest influences were crafting and creating my own closets in the homes I lived in with my mother and father and the valuable insights they passed on to me—my father's tips about clothes and his need for quality and quantity in combination with my mother's penchant for arranging things in a neat and crisp way. All of these experiences fill the pages of this book, which I hope will help you shop your closet. Enjoy!

ACKNOWLEDGMENTS

I thank my family, especially my mother and father, who took such good care of me my entire life, for supporting and encouraging my dreams and aspirations, and my brothers John and Luke for being part of the "triplets" and my best friends. I also thank my friends who supported and encouraged me during this long process, including my literary agent, Stacey Glick; my attorney, Hillary Hughes; Kevin Clark; Keith Geldof; Douglas Friedman; my editor, Anne Cole; and my publishers at HarperCollins. I thank Deborah and Dean Lorich; Burt and Judy Resnick; Christine Schwarzman; Dog Productions; Designer Resale; my In-laws Drs. David Fascitelli and Noel Salem; Mr. and Mrs. Friedman; and Dan Nissanoff. On a special note, many thanks to Caroline Callahan, whose work and vision helped shape the scope of this book. Lastly, I would like to thank my husband, Jon, who has more enthusiasm about everything I do than I do myself and inspires me every day that I am with him. . . . I love you! Thank you, one and all!

INTRODUCTION

The piercing shriek of your alarm clock jolts you awake. Your bare feet touch the cold floor. As you slowly gain consciousness, the age-old question that you face every morning enters your brain: *What am I going to wear?*

While you stumble toward the closet, you think of a great outfit—those fabulous black pants that fit perfectly, maybe a tailored button-down shirt for a uniform look, and your favorite stylish red shoes to add a dash of color—but then you discover that the pants are a wrinkled mess, the shirt is missing buttons . . . and the red shoes? Well, you found the left one, but the right is missing in action. What do you do now?

"What should I wear, and where the hell is it?" is a far more complex issue than most of us are willing to admit. This two-pronged question spawns a host of others: How do you build a wardrobe that won't leave you feeling as if you'd be better off naked? One that allows you easy access to versatile, attractive looks? How do you cultivate a personal style that works for you? And once you have this style and have bought the clothes, how do you organize, store, and preserve them so that they're easy to see and reach?

Shop Your Closet is the answer to all of these questions. It is a go-to guide for all of your concerns about organizing your wardrobe and making your closet an easy, appealing clothes sanctuary. The book is divided into three main sections. The first, "Be Your Own Editor," will instruct you on how to let go of your clothing clutter and maximize and enhance your existing wardrobe. Additionally, it will help you define your personal style and accentuate that style with clothing pieces that may be missing from your existing wardrobe. The second section, "In the Closet," deals with the logistics behind closet organization, helps you decide what organizational tools to buy, and explains how to best use those tools—from hangers to hooks—on a day-to-day basis. Included are tips on how best to store clothing items, from beaded gowns to winter coats, and the debate over whether to hang or to fold is settled once and for all. The third section, "Staying Organized," has guidelines for maintaining your closets on a daily basis and addresses the life-altering question "What do I do when she moves in?" It also provides helpful hints on how to adapt these ideas to other areas of your home, from the medicine chest in your bathroom to the pantry in your kitchen, and looks at problematic storage issues, including CD collections, bookshelves, and seasonal items. A resource guide, helpful hints from fashion industry insiders and leaders, and sidebars give you invaluable information to help you create the closet of your dreams.

Shop Your Closet will inspire you to organize your closets, edit and enhance your wardrobe, and use your storage space to its fullest potential. Unclutter your home, define your personal style, and free yourself from closet nightmares. Turn to chapter 1 and let's begin.

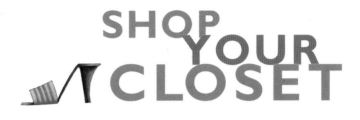

BE YOUR OWN EDITOR

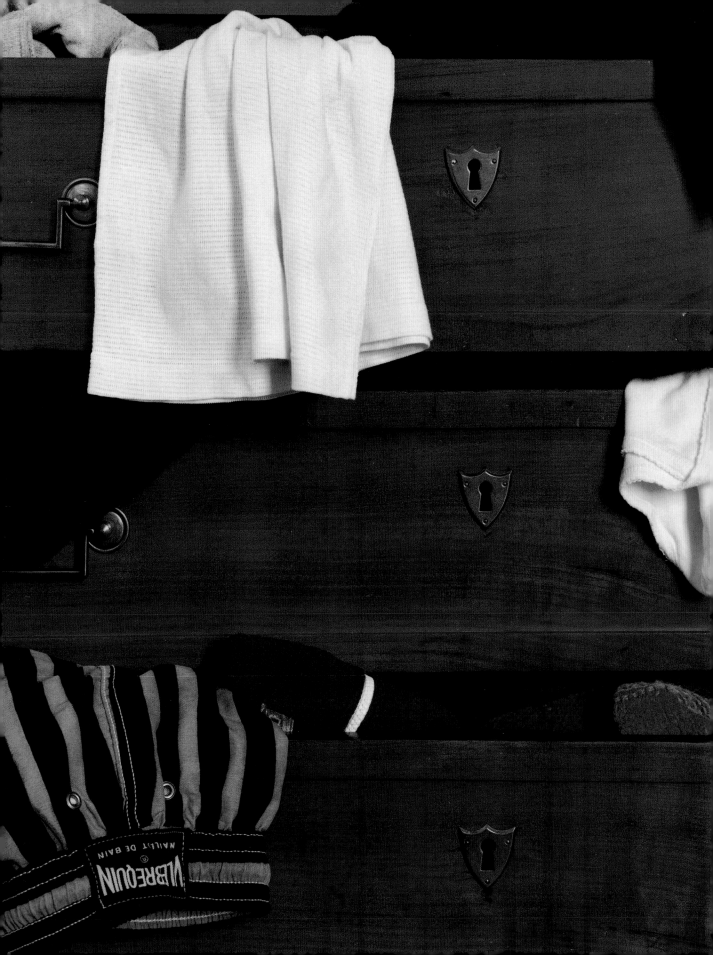

CHAPTER I

Bye-Bye, Pack Rat!

. . . Hello peace of mind.

Most of us share the same embarrassing secret—we hoard. Even the *super*organized among us occasionally hang onto things we don't need—those 24-inch-waist jeans that fit so well three years ago or that dress that you blew your *entire* first paycheck on or the 4-inch-heels (a half size too small!) in purple suede you've never worn but swear you will. The most important step to organizing your closets—and your life—is to lose the habits and ways that make you cling to every little thing. Prior to creating my firm Clos-ette, I have to admit that, yes, even the superorganized me was a pack rat in my other life. I was a bona fide shopaholic who lived to spend every free minute in any type of retail establishment seeking out the latest fashions and hottest clothing trends. When I look back on those days, I think, *Eeew, how vulgar and gross!* That unquenchable desire to seek out the new trends for each season has faded away. Today, I edit my wardrobe every four months and look for things I love to integrate with my wardrobe. I buy classically designed garments that I can keep wearing over and over again. I never grow tired of them, and I change my look by throwing on a great pair of shoes or carrying a new purse. I look good and I feel good. This new way of keeping my closets organized and easy to shop has helped me keep a tighter hold on my wardrobe: I know what I have and I know where it is. And I've discovered that by keeping things neater and more organized in my closet, I have a clearer head when I get dressed to begin my day. I am no longer stressed about where is it, will it be wearable when I find it, and do I have other pieces that will coordinate with it to complete my outfit. I have more important things to ponder. If you have great pieces for each season that fit and are in good condition, and need to buy only a few select items to enhance what you already own, you won't wake up one day and be caught with a closet full of "Oh my God, what the hell is all of this stuff!" clothing and accessories that you just don't wear.

"Purging is a lifelong commitment," says *GQ* creative director Jim Moore, who has been picking and choosing clothes for the magazine since the early 1980s. And any über-organized person will agree: You've got to realize that editing your wardrobe is a constant process. This has never been truer than in today's world, where people are encouraged to buy everything from socks to scarves in bulk.

CHANGING YOUR MIND-SET

The first step to major change is desire. The fact that you picked up this book and got past the table of contents is a good sign that you are willing to take the first steps toward an edited wardrobe and an organized closet. It shows that you want to make your wardrobe a fun place to turn to rather than a space that fills you with anxiety.

The next step toward creating an organized, accessible wardrobe is recognizing that change is possible. Letting go of the pack rat inside you is *definitely* possible; we can assure you of that. Think of the most difficult obstacle you've encountered in your life—a physics class you thought you could never pass, a designer handbag you thought you could never save for, or a huge credit-card bill that you thought you'd never pay off! Whatever the challenge, you were able to face it and overcome it. Similarly, you will be able to stop hanging on to things you don't need.

GETTING STARTED

To get rid of a mess, sometimes you have to make one. Set aside a weekend—or two evenings after work—to review and edit your wardrobe. Remember, your new mantra is *p-u-r-g-e* . Start by sorting your clothes into three categories: "Throw Away," "Give Away," and "Keep." The damaged-beyond-repair—a top that's missing most of its sequins, pants you burned with an iron, anything torn that cannot be repaired—should go into the "Throw Away" pile. No ifs, ands, or buts. The "Give Away" pile should contain anything that's out of style, too small, or (lucky for you!) too big. Donate these items to your local charity shop or clothing drive, consign them to a used-clothing boutique or vintage-clothing store, or give them to a friend. (See chapter 3, "The CDC: Consignment, Donation, and Collecting," for more information on donating versus consigning and the advantages of each.) "The Keep" pile should, of course, contain items that you have worn within the last year and that you will continue to wear.

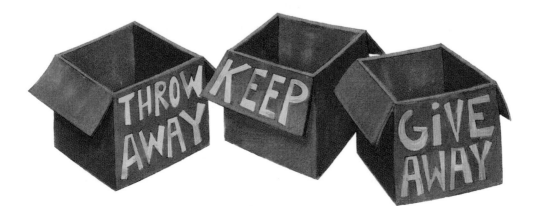

DECONSTRUCTING THE PACKRAT PSYCHE

PACKRAT MANTRA	THOUGHT REPLACEMENT	ADVICE FROM THE PROS
"Just in case."	Out with the old to make room for the new!	Make space to take in new ideas! —AMY ASTLEY, EDITOR, TEEN VOGUE
"What if it comes back in style?"	Make room for what you need now, not what you wore back then.	If you haven't worn it in two years, get rid of it! —WENDY CLURMAN, FORMER VOGUE FASHION DIRECTOR
"I might need this some time down the road."	I probably won't need it, and if I do it can always be replaced.	Sentimentality is bad for the wardrobe. —MIGUELINA, DESIGNER
I'll throw it away later.	Later could mean three weeks, three years, or three decades! Get rid of it now.	Replace "later" with "now" when it comes to the wardrobe. —ALVIN VALLEY, DESIGNER

Sometimes it is difficult to decide what items should be placed in which pile. If this is the case, asking a friend to assist you can help. The key to enlisting a friend-editor is to make certain not to ask anyone who will cause you great emotional duress during this important editing exercise (your brutally honest best friend, your mom, your boyfriend or girlfriend, or anyone else who will make you want to strangle them when they squint their eyes and say, "Hmmm, you look kind of pudgy in that . . ."). Instead, choose a friend who knows your lifestyle and your personality, who you think has good personal style, and who can make sure that you're not going to hang on to an ill-fitting dress just because it's black or you got it on sale.

People cling to clothing and other items for many different reasons, and many think: *Why do I have all this stuff, and how will I be able to let go of it?* The reality is that once you begin to purge your closet of clothing you're not using, you'll be able to think more freely and feel incredibly unburdened by clutter. "Editing my wardrobe is something I have always found very hard," says Emilia Fanjul Pfeifler, president, EF Communications. "Lately, I try not to buy very trendy clothes and instead, I opt for items that work season to season. Generally, if I don't wear something for a year, it has got to go."

CATALOGUE YOUR WARDROBE

Once you've edited sufficiently, take a formal inventory of the items you do have using Clos-ette's inventory sheet as a guide. (Check page 149 of the Resources section at the back of the book for a copy of this sheet.) List all of your sweaters, pants, suits, jackets, outerwear, gym/active wear, dresses, skirts, shoes, and boots by material and color. Although this task may seem a bit daunting, the result is worth the effort—an official, complete inventory of your wardrobe. This will also bring to your attention shopping habits that will need to be addressed: Are you buying too many black turtleneck sweaters or too many button-down shirts? Another benefit will be the emergence of your overall style: Do you own mostly casual or classic clothes and want to be slightly more current with the trends? Or do you tend to purchase more dressy clothes and lack more casual attire? Either way, assessing what you own—and actually writing it down on an ongoing basis—will set you on the right track and keep you organized and wardrobe informed.

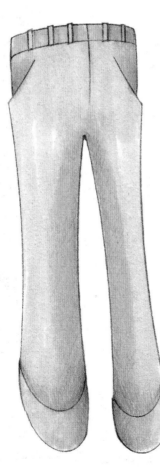

After you've recorded your clothing inventory, decide how to store it and where it will be placed. (For information about storing and specific questions about what should be hung or folded, please refer to chapter 7, "To Hang and to Fold.")

EMOTIONAL TIES

We're not talking men's neckwear here—what we mean is those ties that keep you bound to things that you will most likely never, ever wear. Do you have trouble getting rid of old T-shirts because they remind you of your college days? Or old pairs of jeans because they remind you of a special someone, even when they don't fit? Or a certain bridesmaid's dress from your friend's wedding that maybe you can cut down one day for a cocktail dress? Certain hang-ups (or "hang-ons," in this

top five tips for cleaning out your closet

1. Leave yourself ample time to really review each garment carefully and to complete the task.

2. Have plenty of large trash bags available for throw-away items. Make sure to remove the bags from your home once you've filled them, close them securely, and dispose of them in a proper fashion.

3. Inventory whatever you decide to donate or consign. Make two copies (one for your records and one to include as a packing list with your donation). Make certain that these items are clean and properly packed for easy transportation.

4. Sentimental items, such as christening gowns, wedding dresses, and so forth, should be wrapped in acid-free tissue and archivally stored in an acid-free box. Do not hang sentimental items with your daily wardrobe, as this will cause confusion and may damage your prized heirlooms.

5. Discard all dry cleaner's plastic and plastic bags; don't keep them in your closet.

case) should be eliminated. But if you're prone to intense separation anxiety, allow yourself one or two items to cling to and weed out the others. Sound abstract? Let's take those college tees for a minute: They're beaten up, ratty, some too big, some too small, but you *love* them. The good thing is that T-shirts don't take up a lot of space, so pare your collection down to your favorite four, fold them, and store them in a drawer or on a closet shelf. As you grow more accustomed to the merits of editing your wardrobe, chances are you'll allow yourself to part with them later and enjoy reminiscing about them as you look through photo albums at pictures of you wearing those favorite tees.

And let's face it—many of us simply don't have the space to hang on to large quantities of things we don't wear. I know I don't; my apartment has one minuscule closet. The average urban apartment is usually smaller than the living rooms of our parents' homes in the suburbs and, if we're lucky, contains one very small closet. So unless you're living in a large or huge multiroom apartment complete with more closets and storage space than you could have ever imagined, storing a coat collection, ski pants pile, and a linen stack may cause you a great deal of grief; they just take up so much darn space! Edit those piles. The more realistic you are about your constraints—emotionally and spatially—the more likely you are to establish a successful, useful, and wearable wardrobe.

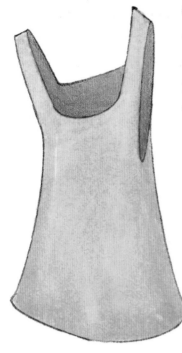

COLOR-CODE AND CATEGORIZE YOUR CLOTHES

Pack rats can't help stashing and hoarding. They make it easier to get away with this by jumbling all their items together rather than sorting clothing by color, type, and season. You know what I mean. It takes the average pack rat 15 minutes to find their favorite white linen shirt because it's balled up underneath their neon-yellow ski suit with the fabulous faux-leopard fur trim they bought on sale while vacationing in Aspen five years ago (which by the way, is two sizes too big and has never been worn—but it was such a bargain!). Group like items together. This will help you mix and match pieces more easily and allow you to do a rapid-fire comparison of what you've got. In this way, if you need a cream-colored silk top to coordinate with your red-and-blue-plaid wool skirt, you can easily find them and pair them.

Organize each category—sweaters, shirts, pants, skirts—from light to dark to further streamline your closet. Now, you will be able to tell at a glance if your favorite red pleated skirt is at the dry cleaner's and not hidden between your navy blazer and pink wide-wale corduroys. Separating clothes by season also makes it easier to locate specific items and allows you to keep tabs on what you have and what you

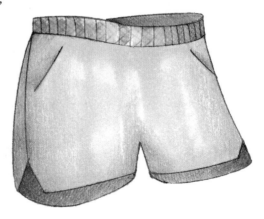

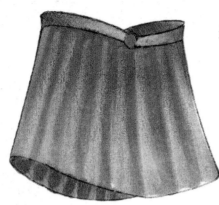

need to replenish or replace. It also makes it easier for you to change your closet from one season to the next, without having to scour your entire home looking for what you will need for the current season.

SPACING OUT

Having trouble figuring out if you've gotten rid of enough things to properly store the wardrobe you are currently wearing? It will be helpful to note these measurements (see next page) to know how much space your various shirts, suits, jackets, skirts, and pants require:

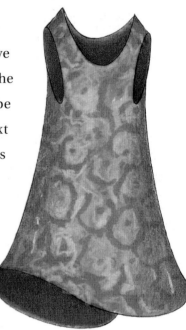

ENDLESS REWARDS

Does all this picking, pitching, and color-coding sound like one huge pain in your neck? Remember that the end result is an orderly, wearable wardrobe that is organized and easy to review. Don't forget to keep a running list of your needs, so that you'll know exactly what to buy before moving on to chapter 2, "Style Counts—Shop Savvy."

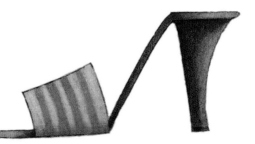

CLOTHING ITEM	WOMEN	MEN	SPACING
Shirts	30–36 inches long	38—49 inches	About 1 inch
Pants	45–52 inches long by cuff or 28–32 inches long folded	51–58 inches long by cuff or 33–38 inches folded	About $1\frac{1}{4}$ –$1\frac{1}{2}$ inches
Jackets and suit jackets	32–42 inches long	39–42 inches	2–$2\frac{1}{2}$ inches
Skirts and dresses	32–44 inches long		$1\frac{1}{2}$ inches; more for pouffy dresses

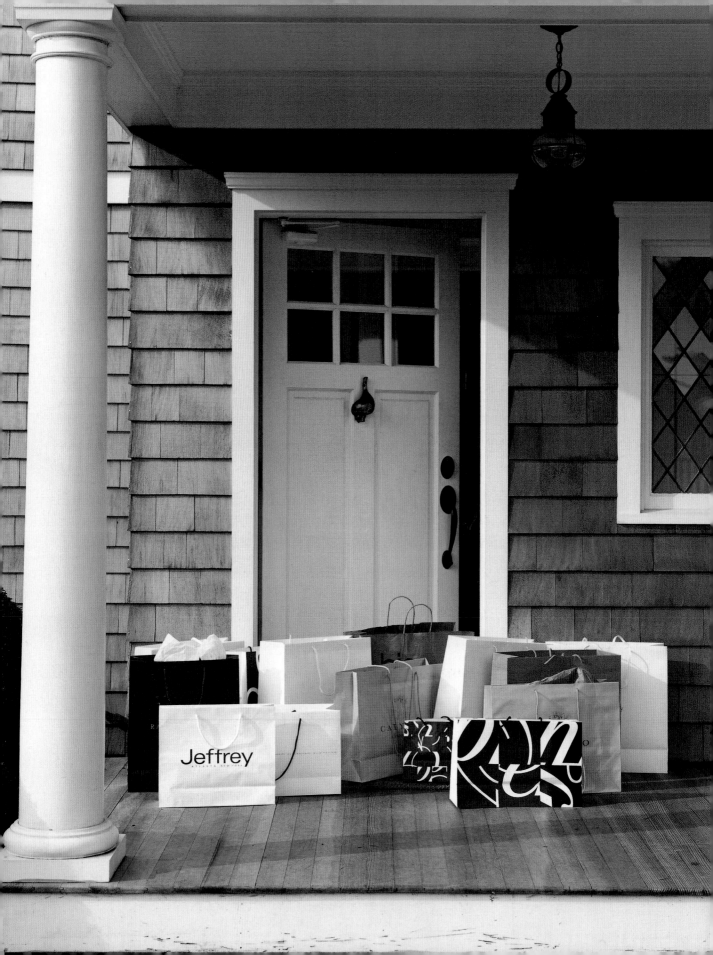

CHAPTER 2

Style Counts— Shop Savvy

I, Melanie Charlton Fascitelli, am a recovering shopaholic. Yes, I admit it, I used to buy for the sheer thrill of buying, and when I would shop I would shop needlessly and wastefully. Now, I buy carefully and think of my entire wardrobe or basic style goals for the season in mind. I hate to admit it, but I just don't have the time to go to my favorite retail haunts. And I will tell you a little secret: I still have a rather zealous shopping streak when it comes to shoes, handbags, and earrings. So what's a girl with no time— who works in a style-centric business—to do? How do you shop with intent and still satisfy the reckless need to accumulate the latest and greatest in the most immediate fashion possible? I shop online, of course. Ah, the Internet. It has brought the world into our homes with a few simple keystrokes or clicks of a mouse. It has become my pathway to the shopping stars, and let me tell you, it is one lean, mean shopping emporium machine! Net-a-porter.com, Shopbop.com, Saksfifthavenue.com, Barneys.com, Vivre.com, Bergdorfgoodman.com, Neimanmarcus.com. My palms are getting sweaty and I am starting to feel lightheaded just thinking about the endless shopping possibilities at my fingertips; I never have to leave my desk chair. This is how I do all of my shopping now. First, I look at the magazines and fashion ads to see what is happening and where it is being sold. I find it online, buy it, and have it shipped. This new way of shopping has streamlined my wardrobe, saves me countless hours and dollars, and prevents me from making impulsive buys. I find that this is a great way to keep myself clothed in both the basics *and* more stylish pieces. My wardrobe and my closet are testaments to my new shopping lifestyle.

You might also be a fan of online shopping, or perhaps you're more of a "bricks and mortar" person, or maybe both. The key is to find out what works for you. Figuring out which method is least stressful for you will leave more time for what's *really* important: picking out a wardrobe that makes you look fabulous!

TAKING STOCK: YOUR PERSONAL FASHION INVENTORY

Okay, you've cleaned out your closet, packed up all the things you want to get rid of, and are now standing in front of your barren closet, feeling a bit empty. What's next? Shopping, of course.

Wait. Before running out the door with credit card in hand ready to pounce on the first bit of clothing to come into your line of vision, be sure you've followed the instructions listed in the previous chapter and have completed your personal fashion inventory (refer to the Resources section at the back of the book for a copy of the inventory sheet). This list will serve as your road map, your personal shopping guide to provide the answers to the top two wardrobe questions: What do I need? What don't I need? It will help you note severe gaps in your wardrobe and figure out what to buy to fill those fashion holes.

A good basic wardrobe consists of pieces that can be mixed and matched to get the best number of wearable combinations to extend the usefulness of

the basic wardrobe

Acclaimed fashion designer Peter Som states that the five basics that should be in every man's wardrobe are black or midnight navy suit, white button-down shirt, white T-shirt, straight-leg dark-rinse jeans, and a pair of black leather brogues. For women: little black dress, white button-down shirt, straight-leg dark-rinse jeans, a great trench coat, and a pair of fabulous heels.

your clothing. Clothes fall into three categories: casual/sport, work/business attire, and evening/special occasion. The following is a rundown of what should be included within each category. The quantity to buy is up to you. Be realistic and buy on the basis of storage space, finances, usefulness, and need. As a working woman (who's also a self-proclaimed shopper and Web-surfing fanatic for all things new and now), I find that my wardrobe has evolved with a strong focus on my business. Because I adore shoes and handbags, they make up about 30 percent. The rest shakes out to be 30 percent dresses, 20 percent jeans, 10 percent tops and shirts, 10 percent sweaters and jackets, 5 percent skirts, and 5 percent suits and slacks. My "uniform" that I usually put on is a classic dress that is one of the staples of my wardrobe, enhanced by a great pair of shoes and a knockout handbag. This works for me and has become my signature style.

Women

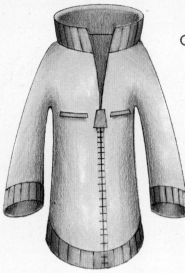

Casual/Sport

* Flattering jeans
* Well-fitting white T-shirts
* Walking shoes/comfortable loafers
* Running shoes/sneakers
* Casual belt to be worn with jeans
* Workout/gym clothing
* Sweaters
* Zipper-front sweatshirt/lightweight jacket

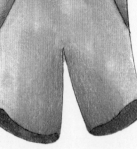

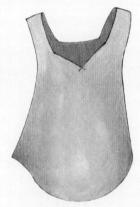

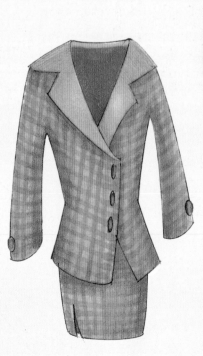

Business/work attire

* Dark business suit in a lightweight wool
* Neutral-colored dress slacks
* White shirts or simple blouses
* Dark-colored belt to coordinate with your shoes

SHOP YOUR CLOSET

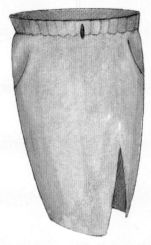

* Neutral-colored/brown belt
* Appropriate business footwear (simple black pumps and a pair of neutral/brown shoes)
* Neutral-colored tailored skirts
* Dark-colored blazer to be worn with skirts or dress slacks
* Winter coat
* Trench coat

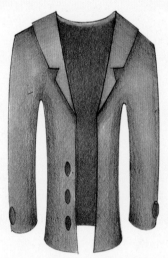

Evening/Special Occasion

* Cocktail dress
* Evening gown
* Evening/dressy heels
* Wrap or shawl

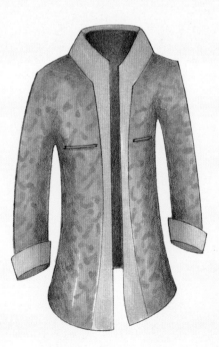

Men

Casual/Sport

* Well-fitting jeans
* T-shirts
* Walking shoes/casual loafers
* Running shoes/sneakers
* Workout/gym gear
* Casual belt to be worn with jeans
* Zipper-front sweatshirt/lightweight jacket
* Sweaters

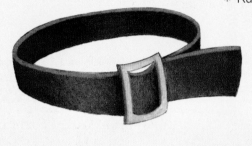

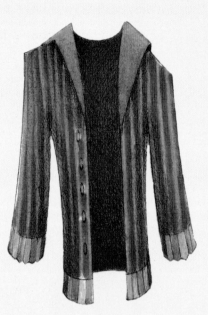

Business/work attire

* Dark-colored suit in lightweight/tropical wool
* Light-colored dress shirts
* Silk ties
* Dark blue blazer
* Neutral-colored dress pants
* Appropriate business footwear with belt to match
* Winter coat
* Rain coat or trench coat

Evening/Special Occasion

* Tuxedo
* Black silk bow tie

KNOW YOUR BODY: WHAT AM I?

Buy clothing that emphasizes your attributes and disguises your flaws. Let's face it: We all have certain parts of our bodies that we would like to play up or play down. Do you have sensational legs? Buy skirts or dresses that show them off. Is your midsection a little bit larger than you would like it to be? Avoid short-waisted tops and sweaters that ride up and emphasize that area of your body. Are you petite and wish you could look a little taller? Choose

SHOPPING AND STYLE ADVICE FROM THE PROS

You have to ruthlessly, brutally assess your style and your whole look, and really know what looks good on you, before you start shopping. Let fashion be your friend.

—Amy Astley, editor, *Teen Vogue*

Seventy-five percent of the evening gowns I wear are borrowed. I am sure there will be a point in my life where I will wish I had invested in more gowns and will find myself, literally, with nothing to wear. But in the meantime, I prefer to spend my money on timeless clothing and quality accessories.

—Lauren Davis, fashion stylist

Personal style is something you have to feel within yourself.

—Miguelina Gambaccini, designer

Go with what people compliment you on!

—Jim Moore, creative director, *GQ*

clothing that visually elongates the vertical lines of your body and avoid busy prints and horizontal patterns. Vertical stripes and similarly colored tops and bottoms give the illusion of an elongated plane, making you appear taller. A black skirt paired with a black turtleneck, providing a continuous solid block of color, will also make you seem taller. Simply put, buy clothes that make you look good. If you don't know what looks good on you, ask a trustworthy, fashion-savvy friend to accompany you on your shopping excursions to provide you with some guidance. As discussed in chapter 1, "Bye-Bye, Pack Rat," do not ask your boyfriend, girlfriend, best friend, mother, or the salesperson who works on commission what they think. Either their answer will enrage you to the point of committing murder (probably theirs) or they won't tell you the truth, leaving you with a closet full of unflattering, unwearable clothing. I've learned to be more honest about what looks good on me. I go with my instincts and listen to the sage advice of those whose opinion I trust. Who wants to have to deal with a bunch of stuff that doesn't look good on them or doesn't fit right? You'll just have to return it to the store it came from or (eek!) keep it and hope that someday it will look good on you. This is just depressing and no fun! So be realistic and go with your instinct and your body. Listen to yourself; you know what works for you. Ninety-nine percent of the time, taking a fashion risk doesn't work for me and is simply a waste of valuable time, money, and effort.

CAMOUFLAGE OR HIGHLIGHT? THE ART OF ENHANCING YOUR ATTRIBUTES AND DISGUISING YOUR FLAWS

When you shop, do you think of your assets and how to best show them off? Do you know what style clothing looks best on you? Do you even know what your assets are? Let's be real. Most people, when they shop for an article of clothing, get lost in the hunt and forget the mission; they focus on what they are looking for rather than who they are shopping for. It's important to remember that for every body type, there is a right and a wrong way to dress. We want our clothes to flatter the fabulous and forgive the flaws. Read on to discover what body type is closest to your figure and how to dress to make the most of what you have.

THE APPLE The apple is full-figured with an undefined waist. The upper portion of the body appears larger than the lower portion, making this body type appear shorter and wider. To best dress for this shape, it's important to bring some definition to the upper body and show off the vertical planes while masking the horizontal area. To accomplish this, avoid wearing tentlike oversized clothing. Baggy shapes provide a lot of room but will emphasize the lack of definition of your body and make you appear larger. Translation: really big clothes make you look really big. Instead, select tops that are a bit more form fitting and that either nip in at the waist or can be slightly belted to give the illusion of a waistline. Also, buy shirts and sweaters that do not cut you off in the middle; they bring attention to the midsection of your body without enhancing its shape, making you look wider and shorter. Instead, select ones with a longer body that hit below the waistline area. This simple fashion trompe l'oeil (which means "fool the eye" in French) results in an unbroken visual plane, making you appear slimmer and taller. Pairing a top in a different shade than your slacks or skirt will also help in defining your waistline.

Avoid large prints, bold colors, and too many details such as sequins, beads, embroidery, ruffles, and excessive pleats. These extras provide too much visual "noise" that detracts from your overall appearance. Pick colors and fabrics that accent your eye and hair color and show off your skin tones. People with darker-toned skin look good in clear, bright colors such as red, blue, and coral. People with ruddy-toned skin look better in colors such as earth tones and deep shades like navy and chocolate brown.

People with yellow-toned skin look better in pale colors such as light blue and pearl pink. To find out which colors work best for you, talk to a fashion consultant (usually available at better retailers or boutiques), see a color specialist at the makeup counter at your favorite department store (they will tell you which colors work best in makeup for your skin tone, hair, and eye color; this information is easily translatable when selecting items for your wardrobe), or visit your local library or search the Internet to discover your personal palette.

When buying pants, choosing a style that is slightly fitted and less baggy. Make sure they aren't too long; it will make you look like you borrowed your big sister's clothing. Also, avoid extremely short or cropped pants. These style slacks, although very trendy, appear as if they shrunk in the dryer and are all-around unflattering. Seek out fabric that is not too bulky or thick. Stay away from anything that's high-waisted. Choose lower-rise pants to make your torso appear longer, giving you a slimmer, more flattering profile.

Skirts should skim the hips and be a little fuller (such as an A-line) toward the hem. This style makes your midsection appear smaller, giving you a nice shape that accents your curves and drawing attention to your defined waist and hips. Overly full styles, such as peasant skirts, are too voluminous and make you look heavier. Remember, the idea is to bring attention to your waistline and hips, not bury them in layers of fabric.

Like certain skirt styles, select dresses that skim your hips and waist area and become fuller toward the hem. The wrap dress, an innovative style in the 1970s that is having a huge renaissance today, is a perfect choice. Avoid trapeze-style dresses or any style that lacks definition. These comfy, roomy garments do nothing to enhance your figure.

THE PEAR Pears are smaller on top and larger in the hips and buttocks. To emphasize the bust and waist, and draw attention away from the lower half of your body, select tops that emphasize your bustline. V-necked sweaters, scoop necked blouses, and shirts with details like ruffles, pleats, embroidery, and beads draw the viewer's eye up and away from your bottom. Wear eye-catching jewelry that shows off your neck and draws attention to your upper torso. A beautiful slightly plunging blouse that shows off a glittering gold chain or strand of drop-dead beads is a knock out!

Pants should be cut more fully and not stretch taut across the butt. Do not wear skin-tight jeans, as they will make your butt look bigger. Avoid embroidered or appliquéd jeans or pants, which will bring attention to your lower half. Dress slacks in neutral dark colors and made out of light-weight fabric will be more flattering to your figure.

Wear skirts and dresses that draw attention to your waist and upper portion of your body. Steer clear of miniskirts or styles with unusual hemlines. These emphasize your lower body and draw people's attention to it. Like "the apple," choose skirts that aren't too full or flouncy. All those extra yards of fabric add bulk and thickness in the wrong places.

THE BANANA The banana body type has an elongated torso and bottom half with hardly any curves. To bring "curve appeal" to your body select clothing that emphasizes the various areas you wish to show off: your bust, your legs, your midriff.

If you're a banana, go with tops that emphasize your bustline and torso. V-necks and fitted shirts with darts and pleats work beautifully to draw the eye to this area of your body. Small patterns, bright colors, and dressmaker details are perfect ways to accent your tops. Do select blouses made of form-flattering fabrics such as silks and knits; these will accentuate curves and highlight your bust. Do not wear oversized shirts or too many layers. This will smooth out any curves you have and give you a boxlike flat-chested appearance. Slight shorter tops that hit at the waistline or slightly above will also bring attention to the upper portion of your body, giving it emphasis and shape.

Choose slacks that highlight your vertical line and skim your hips and buttocks, showing them off to their best potential. Form-fitting jeans and slacks will accent your lower body, giving you eye-catching curves. Wear pants that are long enough to show off your height but not so long that they drag on the ground. Nobody looks good in "street sweepers"; they make you look short and sloppy.

Choose dresses that emphasize your slim figure and your bust. An empire style that is form-fitting to the bust and then sweeps out from the body is an excellent choice. Choose skirts that show off your legs and hips. A shorter skirt with a slightly lower-slung waistline and a bit straighter is a good selection for you.

Now that you know what body type you are, it's time to ponder who you are. What is your personality? How do you want the world to see you? Read on to find out how to put yourself on the world's stage and let everyone know who you are by the way you dress.

KNOW YOUR PERSONALITY: WHO AM I?

Your clothing reflects the type of person you are: fashionable and hip, fun-loving and spirited, serious and focused. It tells the world how you want others to perceive you and what you think of yourself. It's a way of letting people know what they can expect when they encounter you. Your wardrobe is your coat of arms, proudly displaying your personal colors and patterns for the entire world to see. So when you go shopping for pieces to enhance your wardrobe, keep this in mind—you make a statement with what you wear.

FASHIONABLE AND HIP People who are fashionable and hip know what's hot and what's not. They read all the latest fashion magazines; can tell you what every star wore to the Oscars, Emmys, and Tonys (and which designers made each gown); and follow religiously what is being shown on the runways in Milan, Paris, and New York. They know where to shop to get the latest fashion, and their closets reflect current trends in style, fabric, color, silhouette, and detail. Their wardrobe changes a lot, and they would never wear anything "last season."

FUN-LOVING AND SPIRITED People who are fun-loving and spirited select clothes that enhance and proclaim their passion for what they do, whether it's rock climbing, horseback riding, or golf. Bright colors, eye-catching patterns, and styles that fit their lifestyle predominate. They aren't afraid to be noticed, and they aren't shy. A touch of whimsy and accessories that show off their distinct personality become their trademark. Their wardrobe is a reflection of their personality and passion for life.

SERIOUS AND FOCUSED People who are serious and focused select classically designed, no-nonsense clothing that provides the most efficient service and wear. Their wardrobe shuns trends and loud colors, as they do not want to draw attention to themselves. Their clothing is a part of their total personality and is worn because it needs to provide cover, warmth, and the ability to function within society. Their few good, basic pieces are easily mixed and matched, and nothing frivolous or superfluous exists in their closet.

SHOPPING FOR YOUR PERSONALITY

When you're building and maintaining a wardrobe, it's easy to fall into a rut. No matter how many great options there are out there, most of us tend to buy clothing that falls into certain patterns. You know what I mean. Do you keep buying that almost identical little black dress every time you need a special outfit for that amazing event coming up? Or when you shop for a new business outfit, do you pick up yet again another pants-and-blazer combination of charcoal gray lightweight wool pinstripe fabric where the slacks have a slightly flared leg and the jacket is double-breasted just like the other nine suits hanging in your closet? Open that door, look inside, and visually dissect your wardrobe; review the clothes hanging in your closet and notice the distinctive pattern that emerges. Does a certain color predominate? How many black shirts and sweaters do you have? Do specific styles or types of clothing seem to fill your shelves and racks? Is there a sea of business attire and little casual wear? Does your shoe collection threaten to overtake your entire apartment?

The simplest way to break these patterns is by following these two basic steps: (1) inventory and catalogue your wardrobe as we discussed earlier in chapter 1, "Bye-Bye, Pack Rat," and (2) when you shop, consciously look for fashion that is outside your comfort zone. If you never wear color (you wear only black, white, or gray) look at pieces in blue, earth tones, or—gasp . . . dare I say it?—red. If you always buy classically styled clothing, look at things that are a bit more trendy to spice up and update your wardrobe. If you tend to always buy casual clothing, stray into the evening-wear section of your favorite store and try on some elegant cocktail dresses or a sensual pair of black satin evening pants with a sparkly, beaded top. These two easy steps can change your shopping patterns and breathe new life and diversity into your closet.

Now, we are all a bit like Sybil (remember the book where many distinctive personalities inhabited one woman) in that we have many moods and dress according to how we feel on a particular day. For example, suppose it's Monday, it's raining, and you have three meetings and a really long conference call in the afternoon. You know you will *never* get a taxi on a day like this and you're running late. What do you put on? Of course, you wear the standard black pantsuit that never wrinkles, requires little conscious thought, is water repellant, and matches your mood and the weather outside your window. But wait—let's rewind and look in your closet again. Don't buy into that murky spell cast by the rain and your crowded work calendar; put on your favorite red skirt with that great patterned tailored shirt and dispel the gloom Or if you don't have the time to change, throw on a wildly patterned scarf or a piece of colorful jewelry to add a splash of personality to your ensemble. By simply perking up your outfit, you may lift your mood and change your approach to the entire day!

I know we are all creatures of habit and buy what we like and feel comfortable or secure wearing. But it's time to mix it up and break some of these fashion patterns and moods. Here are some ideas on how to expand your shopping horizons and what to buy to enhance your wardrobe, while allowing yourself the opportunity to explore some other personalities.

Think Small

To start making personality and pattern changes in your wardrobe, begin by taking small steps. Start by selecting a colored, patterned shirt if you normally wear a neutrally colored solid. Buy a trendy skirt to add a little touch of whimsy to your casual collection. Pick up a pair of great shoes in a color you would never buy, such as emerald green, to give your favorite party frock a new look. Start small and choose accessories—jewelry, shoes, handbags, scarves, and belts—that add a little zing to your outfits, without breaking the bank or disrupting your personal essence. Sometimes, a new outlook on fashion can begin with the purchase of a trendy hot pink belt to add a color splash to your normally conservative look.

Think Seasonally

When expanding your fashion horizons, use your seasonal needs as a way to explore uncharted territory. If you find out that you've made a wrong choice or a so-so selection or if you wish to explore another style or personality, you can easily give the item to a friend, consign it, or donate it at the end of the season. (See the next chapter: "The CDC: Consignment, Donation, and Collecting".)

WINTER Short, stark, cold days. Long, frosty, crystal-clear nights. Snow and ice. Winter is a great season to explore new colors and designs for your wardrobe. Cold-weather accessories such as hats, gloves, scarves, and earmuffs provide a terrific opportunity to check out the hottest colors, latest materials, and fabulous new patterns to add a spark to these dark, cold days. A colorful scarf combined with a sassy knit hat and a great pair of cashmere gloves can turn your ho-hum serviceable wool overcoat into a show-stopping winter outerwear ensemble. A great pair of boots, worn with jeans, pants, skirts, or dresses, can metamorphose your seasonal office apparel in the blink of an eye. Even the simplest of changes, such as a vintage brooch pinned on to your lapel or the brim of your hat, can add a touch of seasonal festivity and transform your serviceable cold-weather wardrobe into winter finery. Purchasing a new wool skirt in a vivid hue, a cashmere turtleneck in an unusual knit, or a ski jacket in an eye-catching shade lifts your mood and infuses your personal look with a jolt of style.

SPRING Flowers are blooming. The days are getting warmer. This wonderful time of the year is a reawakening, a rebirth of the Earth where everything begins to green and flower. Spring provides the perfect opportunity to add a sense of new life and freshness to your wardrobe. Pick out a top in a beautiful feminine floral pattern to add color and a touch of softness to a pair of dark dress slacks. Buy a beautiful dress in a pale pastel to wear for special nights out. Choose accessories that transform the neutral-tone pieces in your closet into harbingers of the season. Look for fun earrings, playful necklaces, and cheery bracelets to lighten the mood and add a touch of frivolity.

SUMMER Ah, summer! The beach, warm breezes, long sun-filled days, and warm star-filled nights are trademarks of this amazing time of year. To welcome this season of seasons, buy one killer blouse that you can wear to an outdoor concert in the park, on casual Fridays at the office, or on a weekend getaway in the mountains or at the shore. Pick up a dressy tank in a bright shade to show off your tan that can be worn under a jacket to the office or paired with a pair of shorts for a Saturday barbeque. Buy a bathing suit or two in great summery shades that show off your figure and skin tone. A strappy pair of white sandals, a pair of way-cool sunglasses, and a straw bag can transform your everyday clothes into a fresh, carefree resort look. Special note: flipflops are great for the weekend and for casual wear, but please never consider them as serious footwear for the office. That just looks tacky!

FALL The season of brilliantly hued leaves, cool crisp days, chilly nights, fall brings the chance to put on sweaters. Embrace this season and buy a gorgeous wrap to wear when going out for a late dinner or stroll, a cozy cashmere sweater in an eye-popping autumnal shade of russet or saffron, or a pair of comfortable corduroys in a rich jewel-tone color such as topaz or sapphire and pair them with your favorite sweaters or tops. Here's the perfect opportunity to buy a beautiful tweed skirt in heather tones or a pair of wool slacks in camel or tan in a handsome English wool. These classics can be dressed up or down depending on need, and they never lose their appeal.

Think Globally

One of the best ways to add personality to your wardrobe is to look outside of your neighborhood, town, city, or country for fashion inspiration. Like every great designer, you can be inspired by what you see in the movies, read in books and magazines, get from the news, and observe when traveling on vacation or for business. Notice color pairings, fabric choices, patterns, details, and style. Embrace these rich experiences and translate them into your wardrobe. A fantastic embroidered belt from Africa can enliven your Saturday standard jeans-and-white-shirt outfit by giving it a touch of pattern and color. A length of silk sari from India can be used as a gorgeous evening wrap to add glamour to your little black dress when worn for a special office function or elegant dinner party. A chunky, ethnically inspired bracelet from South America lends personality to a business suit. A hand-knit wool scarf in your favorite club colors from England give your winter coat a dash of style and flair. You don't need a ton of these things to make an impact. One or two well-selected pieces will give your wardrobe a distinctive personal touch that is uniquely and singularly you.

who are you, and what's in your closet?

The Life of the Party Oh sure, she has everyday clothes, such as jeans, button-down shirts, and crewneck sweaters, but the life-of-the-party gal lives for the nightlife. Cocktail dresses from Armani, Dolce & Gabbana, and Gucci seductively whisper as you rustle through them to see what's hanging in her closet. Rows of drop-dead gorgeous shoes by Jimmy Choo, Prada, and Manolo Blahnik peek from their racks at the bottom of the closet, while Judith Lieber and Chanel evening bags sit patiently on their shelf waiting to be taken to the next black-tie event. Sparkling costume jewelry glistens like stars on a cloudless night from their black velvet trays, and silk scarves and evening wraps wave like the racing flags on luxury yachts, beckoning to be worn. Business clothing takes a backseat to her finery. Whenever she shops, she always is thinking about the perfect outfit to wear on her next night on the town.

The Business Executive The no-nonsense business executive focuses on her career and her business wardrobe. Rows of freshly dry-cleaned, classically styled business suits in varying shades of navy, charcoal gray, and black hang in perfect symmetry by designer, including Ralph Lauren, Yves Saint-Laurent, and Anna Sui. Tailored shirts in the palest of pastels and whites are freshly laundered and starched, waiting to be worn to that next all-important meeting. Simple pumps in black, navy, and dark brown are freshly polished and lined up on their rack, segregated by color and style. Simple gold jewelry carefully organized in a drawer, complete with jewelry dividers, can be worn with any of her suits. Her one all-purpose, always-in-style little black dress hangs in the back of the closet, waiting to be worn to the next office function.

The Too-Busy Mom The super-busy, carpooling, handle-a-million-tasks-a-day woman focuses on her family. Rows of clean khakis and jeans hang from their hangers, waiting to be jumped into at a moment's notice. Easy-to-care-for, hassle-free shirts and tops from the Banana Republic, Talbots, Lands' End, L.L. Bean, and Brooks Brothers, in many colors, hang in their spot waiting to be paired up with her favorite sweater or pullover. Rows of comfortable, gotta-get-things-done shoes and sandals are lined up in the bottom of the closet, waiting for their next trip to town. Flouncy skirts, flirty tops, and party clothes hang in the back of the closet for special occasions and weekend dinner parties with friends.

The Fitness Diva Even though she has a career and a social life, this gym devotee focuses on her true passion: exercise. Rows of warm-up suits hang in perfect pairs, waiting to be taken out for a run. Gym shorts, tank tops, sports bras, T-shirts, and leotards are perfectly folded on shelves ready for the next kickboxing class. All different types of specialty sneakers and exercise footwear are racked and poised, ready to go. Her business suits, evening clothes, and casual hang-around-the-house clothing fill the rest of her closet.

The All-Arounder The all-arounder has many interests and many moods, and her closet is a peek into her world. There are stored outfits for every occasion and circumstance, ranging from the most formal of events (a great designer gown or two hangs in her closet) to a picnic at the beach (a perfect cotton short set from the Gap sits ready). Business suits hang next to party clothes and cocktail dresses, and workout clothes, casual outfits, and shirts intermingle with dress slacks, jeans, and blazers. Her shoe rack contains everything from her splurge pair of evening heels to her walk-around Tod's. The rest of the space is filled with sneakers, sandals, clogs, and business shoes.

PREPARING FOR BATTLE: HOW TO PLAN, WHAT TO WEAR, AND WHAT TO BRING ON YOUR SHOPPING SPREE

DECIDE WHERE YOU WANT TO SHOP Would you like to check out some fabulous boutiques? Do you feel the urge to visit your favorite department store? Is the siren song of the mall calling to you from the suburbs? Are you dying to hit the outlet stores and see what types of bargains you can snatch up? Whichever options you choose, make a game plan and allow yourself enough time to successfully shop for the things that you need. Also, be certain that you have enough cash and/or the appropriate debit and credit cards with you to make your shopping trip as stress-free as possible.

GIVE YOURSELF PLENTY OF TIME A hurried excursion to the store can leave you with unwanted, inappropriate, ill-fitting items that will end up languishing in your closet with the tags still dangling from them. Let's face it no matter what the size on the label, each manufacturer has its own interpretation of size that can vary wildly from garment to garment. That size small Banana Republic shirt that you love might be absolutely huge and swimming on you, while the size small shirt from Abercrombie & Fitch barely fits across your shoulders and you can't even button it! Take the time to selectively review the clothing at a particular store, and most importantly, try each piece on.

DRESS COMFORTABLY Wear clothing that can easily be taken off and put back on again so that you can try on potential purchases with as little aggravation as possible. No one wants to have to waste precious time struggling out of layers of clothing and wrestling them back with each trip to a dressing room. Do not wear your leotard with a wool turtleneck and bulky cardigan over your favorite pair of leggings, paired with your dashing tartan kilt. Remember, you will not purchase anything that you have not tried on (excluding packaged socks and underwear).

BRING THE RIGHT ITEMS WHEN LOOKING FOR SPECIFIC CLOTHING PIECES If you are shopping for an evening dress, always bring along a pair of heels and a strapless bra to be able to get an accurate idea of how it looks on you. In this way, you can be completely certain that the dress you are trying on is truly a good fit. This will help you avoid making costly fashion mistakes that end up as unworn clutter in your closet.

BRING ALONG A SNACK AND SOME WATER Hunger and thirst can be terribly distracting when you are shopping for clothes and can cause you to make some rash decisions. But avoid any snacks that can be too messy, such as candy bars and chips. No one wants to purchase any clothes with food stains on them.

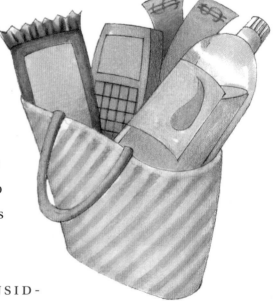

MANNERS COUNT; BE CONSIDERATE If you try something on and it doesn't fit, return the item to its hanger, properly hung, and bring it to the dressing-room attendant or back to the rack where you found it. Don't leave anything in a heap on the floor or flung into a pile at the back of the dressing room. Nobody wants to try on a wrinkled or stained garment.

BE PATIENT Sometimes you may not find exactly what you want immediately on entering your favorite boutique or department store. Take the time to look. Be critical. Carefully examine the piece before trying it on. Be savvy. Find out when your usual shopping haunts or a boutique you have always wanted to visit but never have is having a sale. Search the Internet to find stores near you that carry your favorite designers; check the local newspapers for advertised sales; read your favorite magazines for hot new places to shop; network with friends to find out about sample sales at showrooms or trunk shows at their favorite haunts. And above all else, do not wait until the day before a major business meeting or social event to find that perfect suit or that stunning evening dress. Chances are you will end up settling for an outfit that is less than stellar, that will end up in a heap at the bottom of your closet!

QUALITY VERSUS QUANTITY, OR THE BEST VERSUS THE MOST

When buying a major piece of clothing for your wardrobe—a winter coat, that all-important business suit, the classic navy blazer that will go with everything—buy the best that you can afford. A well-constructed garment of fine material will, with proper care and maintenance, last longer and be more likely to retain the best aspects of its appearance than a cheaper version crafted of lesser-quality material. Let's say you are in the market for a new cardigan. At the store there is a wonderful selection of yummy cashmere sweaters. The feel, the graceful drape, the attention to detail, the style, the way it is knit, and the cut are breathtaking, and there is a price tag to match. In the same store, there is a tremendous selection of synthetic-blend sweaters. They're okay, but they don't feel as nice as their cashmere cousins; the quality of craftsmanship is not there, and the fabric is made of some unknown manmade fiber that you have never heard of or can even pronounce. But the price is less than half that of the cashmere models. What should you do? The old expression "You get what you pay for" truly does apply. One well-selected, high-quality item will last 10 times longer than the cheaper counterpart. The person who buys wisely and well will always have something to wear. The individual who buys volumes of substandard garments will always struggle with the often-heard complaint "I've got nothing to wear." Shop wisely. Shop thoughtfully. The end result will be a wardrobe that truly reflects who you are.

Now that you have purchased your new clothing and your wardrobe is fairly complete, read the next chapter, "The CDC: Consignment, Donation, and Collecting," to find out which option is right for the stuff you want to get rid of.

renting

versus

buying

A new trend that is becoming more prevalent is renting dresses and gowns for special occasions instead of buying them. Renting gives the wearer an opportunity to try something new, to dress in a vintage gown that is not readily available to buy, or to step out in a fabulous designer creation without having to shell out a great deal of money for one occasion. Or in the case of those who must attend numerous social and charitable events during the year, it allows them the freedom to wear a number of different things without cluttering up their closets. Neva Lindner, founder of Wardrobe NYC notes, "I am surprised by how many socialites I work with. It is simply cost-effective to rent sometimes. If you go to four or five events per week and are going to be photographed, a socialite may want to mix it up a bit, perhaps buying one piece, borrowing one piece, and renting one piece. Furthermore, not all socialites are simply able to borrow; it is a privilege available to a selected few." She further says that if someone truly loves a piece and wants to own it, of course she buys it. She continues, "However, there is less and less stigma to renting. You can rent anything from a villa in the south of France to a private jet. It is just as luxurious to come to my loft, have a glass of wine, and choose something for an event as it is to buy. And when they are done with the piece, they don't have to worry about storing it if it is never to be worn again. Closet space in New York City is at a premium."

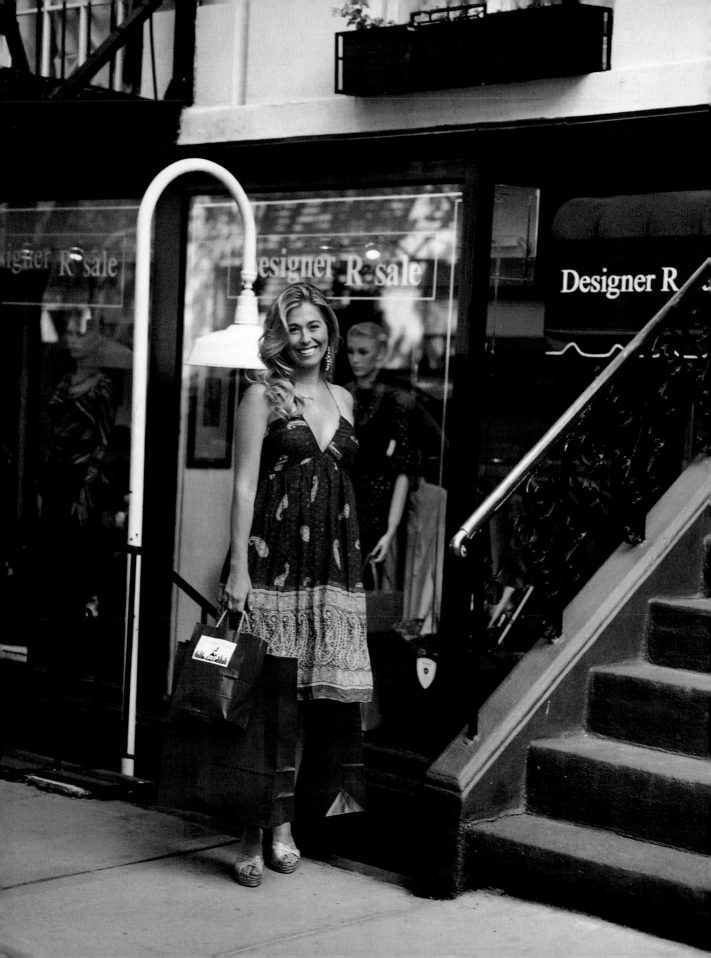

CHAPTER 3

The CDC: Consignment, Donation, and Collecting

The closet is clean. Your new things are ready to be put away. Yet you still have bags and bags of unwanted clothes in your home. What do you do with them? Do you donate them to your favorite charity? Give them away to your friends? Consign them at your favorite resale boutique? Bring them to a vintage clothing or costume shop for them to sell? Put them on eBay (or hand them off to a company that will put them on eBay) and become an Internet retail–auction entrepreneur? Host a house or garage sale? Or if the item is truly valuable and is representative of a known designer, such as an original Bob Mackie beaded dress from the 1970s or a Balenciaga gown from the 1950s, do you save it and start (or add it to) an existing collection? Don't fret! Read on to find out which route is right for you. I learned firsthand about reselling my stuff in college. This helped defray the cost of my shopping, saved me space in my small dorm room, and cleared my social karma of the typical American consumer need for accumulation.

TO CONSIGN OR NOT TO CONSIGN?
THAT IS THE QUESTION

You've gone through everything you want to get rid of, and the first thing that comes to mind is *Where do I take all this stuff?* If you followed the directions from chapter 1, "Bye-Bye, Pack Rat," the damaged and unsalvageable has been tossed and the remainder—good, usable clothing that someone else can wear—is neatly folded and ready to be transported. Decide if you want to consign it, sell it on eBay, or donate it to a thrift shop. Each one of these options has its benefits and drawbacks that are discussed in this chapter.

A consignment shop is a retailer that sells clothing items that have been consigned to the store by an individual. Some prefer to handle only designer or high-end clothing, while others will accept any clothing as long as it is in excellent condition and can be resold. In the past, consigning clothing or shopping at a consignment shop had a negative connotation, a sort of "classless" label associated with it. Many felt that it was what people without means did to get money to pad their incomes or purchase something of quality that they would *never* be able to afford at a regular retailer. Times have changed, and today, even those with considerable means (billionaires included) enjoy shopping consignment stores and receive a tremendous amount of empowerment from reselling their high-end purchases when they are no longer wearing them.

I learned firsthand about consignment shops after I graduated from New York University and landed my first couple of fashion-related jobs. The consignment shops allowed me to sell pieces that I was no longer wearing and let me buy new things at a reduced price from regular retail (such as that next great Prada bag or pair of designer shoes), letting me support my shopping habit without breaking the bank or filling my closets with tons and tons of clothes. It also gave me a sense of excitement in getting money back from something that I had purchased earlier. I know I didn't get a lot of money for my stuff (probably close to 30 percent of the original price). But I looked at it this way: I wore it, I loved it, I was ready to move it along to the next person. So before you load up the car and start driving around town, establish a game plan and chart your course of action for your consignment trek. I did, and it saved me a lot of time, aggravation, and stress and gave me great monetary rewards.

The first step is to "let your fingers do the walking" and consult your local telephone directory, drawing up a list of viable resale/consignment clothing stores in your area. Or if you're computer savvy, search the Internet to get the names of local places that are nearby and look interesting. This list will be your personal consignment guide and a good beginning, but before you run out the door and go to the nearest shop to drop your clothing, do your homework. Visit the stores and see what type of clothing they sell. Look at the merchandise. Are they loaded up with Armani suits and Manolo Blahniks? Or does their inventory show a lot of Anne Klein dresses, casual sportswear from the Gap and Old Navy, and Easy Spirit pumps? Ask the manager or a sales associate about how they consign and what percentage of the sale price they keep. Many consignment shops work on a 50-50 split. However, there is no standard rule, so find out what their policy is. Don't be afraid to negotiate. The worst thing that could happen is the store could say no and you're on to the next name on your list. During your conversation, ask them what types of garments they prefer to retail and if they favor any one designer or designers. Ask how much clothing they'll accept from one consignee and if they work on a seasonal schedule. (In other words, will they take your old winter coat on consignment in May, or do you have to wait until September to bring it in?) Find out what they do with unsold clothing: Do they donate it to a reputable charity and provide you with the receipt? Throw it away or give it away? Sell it to a clothing converter and have it made into rags? Or do they make you pick it up and haul it back to your home? Ask how long they'll try to sell your items and how they pay their consignees (that's you) when items are sold. Finally, don't forget to check with the Better Business Bureau or your local chamber of commerce to see if anyone has filed complaints against them. Now, you're ready for the next step.

You've selected the consignment shop that you think will meet your needs. You know they love handbags and you have 50 in excellent condition that are dying to be resold! (You have your eye on a new beauty or two from Dolce & Gabbana that is screaming to be part of your collection.) And you've negotiated the most amazing 90-10 split that will guarantee you big bucks if the stuff sells. Now it's time to get the goods in order. Make a complete inventory of the items you're going to consign with the shop. Don't forget to include a description of each article of clothing, the designer's name (if applicable), the overall condition of the garment, and a reasonable amount that you would like your item to sell for. A basic rule is to ask approximately half of what you paid for the garment. If you're not sure what to ask in terms of price, check with the store for guidance. Check each piece to make sure it's clean and in good repair. (Nobody wants to buy anything that is torn, damaged, or stained, unless you own an item of major historical/cultural significance and importance—Marie Antoinette's petticoat, Betsy Ross's sewing cap, Marilyn Monroe's notorious white dress, Dorothy's ruby slippers, and so forth. In this case, do not consign the garment. Bring it to your local museum with the associated proof of provenance and let them guide you as to your best course of action.) Fold or hang the clothing neatly to avoid wrinkling and creasing, and pack the items in garment bags, shopping bags, suitcases, or boxes. When you deliver it to the designer/general resale shop, have the person receiving your things sign your inventory list and keep a copy (of the signed one, of course!). This is your personal documentation of what they have and in what condition you delivered it to them. Don't be surprised if the store asks you to sign their contract or personal agreement. If there is anything you don't agree with or understand, do not sign it! Once you do, you are legally obligated to follow the directives outlined in the document. Instead, take your stuff to a different consignor. Finally, don't forget to check the pockets of the items you're consigning to make sure they are empty. No one wants to give away prescription eyeglasses, designer sunglasses, a current passport, a credit card, a piece of jewelry, wads of cash, or a small fortune in change. On the other hand, no one wants to buy an article of clothing with pockets filled with dirty tissues, gum wrappers, lint bunnies, or pieces of paper.

Vintage clothing can be consigned to a designer or general resale store, but most retailers who specialize in antique or vintage clothing usually carry only those types of garments. Do not confuse the two: vintage/antique clothing shops sell garments that are of a period; designer resale shops sell designer clothing. Many vintage/antique clothing retailers consign in a manner similar to that of designer/general resale stores, while others purchase outright the garments they're offered, because of the delicate nature and condition of the merchandise they offer for sale. No matter how the store acquires its inventory, make sure that you're satisfied with the terms that you've worked out with them.

eBAY, BABY!

The Internet retail/auction phenomenon, eBay being the most famous and well known, is another way for you to sell excess clothes. However, unless you work with an authorized eBay outlet, you're responsible for registering, writing accurate descriptions, photographing each item, posting items, setting up payment, and handling all shipping, insurance, and returns yourself. It's not a difficult task, but it is an involved one.

tips for buying and selling fashion online

Before buying or selling anything online, check to make sure you understand the various rules and regulations that must be followed on whatever online retail/auction Web site you choose. If you're unclear on anything, contact the company to get your questions answered before moving forward. A little bit of homework and fact-gathering can save you a lot of headaches and confusion.

Daniel Nissanoff, author of the book *Futureshop: How the New Auction Culture Will Revolutionize the Way We Buy, Sell, and Get the Things We Really Want* (www. futureshopbook.com), lists the following helpful hints when buying or selling fashion online:

Buying

* The old adage "Caveat emptor" ("Let the buyer beware") applies every time. If the deal is too good, the merchandise may be fake. Use sites such as Portero .com instead of eBay to ensure authenticity of an item.
* Purchase expensive items only from reputable sellers. Avoid anyone with less than 97 percent positive feedback.
* Make sure you know your size in the brand you are buying and that the item for sale has not been altered. Many of these Web sites have a no-return policy or one that is very strict. So make sure you know what it is you are buying and that it will fit before you buy it.

* Less is more. Because things are less expensive online, people tend to buy a lot more than they would normally offline. Don't get carried away; just buy what you absolutely love.

Selling

* Stick with nationally recognized brands. It won't sell well unless the brand or designer is recognized in Kansas (even if all the socialites in New York City wear it!).

* Use eBay drop-off stores for accessories such as handbags and shoes. In general, they will get better prices for you than consignment stores will because they will get better visibility.

* Get rid of your stuff as soon as you fall out of love. Don't wait to sell your things thinking that you may eventually wear them again someday. The longer you wait, the less desirable your fashion item will be, and in turn, the less money you will get for it when you finally go to sell it.

* If you've never worn a garment or accessory and can return it to a nationally recognized retailer for credit, you can sell the credit for more money than you can sell the actual item. There is a big market for store credit on eBay.

THE JOYS OF DONATING

Donating clothing is a terrific and simple way to quickly and easily rid your home of piles of stuff. There are many reputable charities that accept clothing donations for various causes, such as One World Running, Dress for Success, and American Red Cross Disaster Services. Some have actual retail outlets or thrift shops that accept clothing contributions, such as Goodwill, the Salvation Army, and the Society of St. Vincent de Paul. Before dropping anything off, contact the organization and ask what types of restrictions apply and how to donate to their charity; each organization has its own procedures and rules regarding donations. And many organizations provide free pickup from your home, such as the Vietnam Veterans of America, which will send a truck to pick up your donations of clothing and other household items.

When donating clothing to a recognized charity, you can claim these donations as deductions from your taxes. Don't forget to get a receipt for your donation from the organization or a letter stating that no goods or services were provided in return for your donation, and submit this information to your accountant or tax preparer. (Note: donation restrictions do apply and deductions can only be taken up to $5,000. If you donate more than $5,000 of any one type of item, you must file form 8283 with the Internal Revenue Service, complete with an appraisal from a licensed appraiser stating the value of the clothing or goods that you have donated for a specific calendar year. If you're unclear on what to deduct for your donations, confer with your accountant or tax preparer.)

COLLECTING CLOTHING—COMPLICATED OR COMPELLING?

Collecting is a great way to hold onto that fabulous Givenchy coat, the timeless Yves Saint-Laurent cocktail dress you know you'll never be able to replace, or that original Hermès Kelly bag. However, when you collect—clothing, furniture, decorative objects, artwork, stamps, coins, or whatever—you assume a responsibility for the maintenance of each item, so that its value and prestige will be retained. That fabulous Oscar de la Renta dress is worth only how well it is preserved and the condition it's kept in. Like fine antiques, such as porcelain and furniture, condition and rarity determine value (not to mention appeal and current popular tastes and trends in the marketplace). And the ultimate thing to consider when you start a collection is: Do I have the space to collect it?

Storage Preservation Tips for Specific Clothing

Whether you're collecting or simply want to take care of that special garment, make sure to store it properly to keep it in the best condition possible. Invited last minute to a fabulous New Year's Eve soirée? You'll want that vintage beaded cocktail dress in tip-top condition. Romantic night with the boyfriend? That pure-silk nightie should be wrinkle-free and gorgeous. Here are some tips to make sure everything is ready and perfect at a moment's notice.

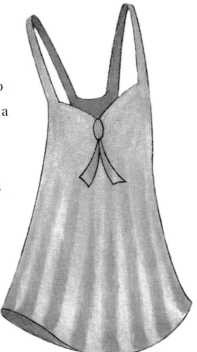

DELICATES/SILKS Delicates and silks should be stored lying flat on sheets of acid-free tissue paper to prevent damage and protect the garments from bleeding. (To purchase acid-free tissue paper, check with your favorite home furnishings store or your local paper goods retailer.) Folding these items can cause permanent creases in the individual garment and may be unremovable. Hanging is not recommended, as the items slip easily off hangers and their lightweight fabric makes it easy for them to get tangled up and twisted among other garments.

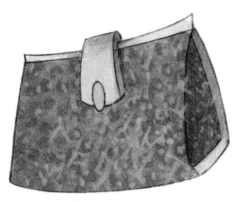

BEADED/SEQUINED ITEMS Pieces that are beaded or sequined can be difficult to store for two reasons: They tend to be very heavy, and the beadwork/sequins can catch on other garments and cause snags, tears, or loss of beading. To store, carefully lay these items on sheets of acid-free tissue and store as you would delicates/ silks. For more detailed information, please refer to Chapter 5, *"To Hang and to Fold "* (page 73).

FURS Climate control is the mantra for fur storage. Never store your furs in plastic. Customized climate-controlled closets can be installed in your home for fur storage, but they are fairly costly. A good alternative is to check your local phone directory or search the Internet to find local furriers or cleaning establishments that offer cold storage for your fur pieces. Prices can vary greatly, as can the cost of insurance coverage and liability in case your items are lost, damaged, or stolen. So be certain to check out establishments carefully before you leave anything in their care.

SPECIAL HATS/SHOES When you purchased your special hat, it probably came in a specific box that was designed to hold it. This is one of the cases in which it's good to hold on to the packaging; use that specific hatbox to store your hat. These boxes are usually constructed of stiff cardboard that prevents crushing of the contents. You can also wad sheets of acid-free tissue paper and put them in the bowl of the hat to help keep its shape. Never store special hats in plastic bags or in piles on shelves. Special shoes usually come with individual shoe bags for storage. Save these bags and use them. Shoe trees are great for maintaining the shape of your shoes in storage. Never put shoes away wet or dirty, as they can crack, mildew, or stain.

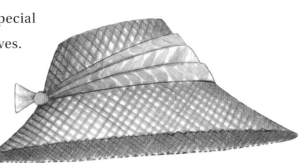

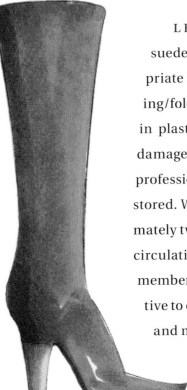

LEATHER/SUEDE Leather and suede items should be stored on appropriate heavy-duty hangers to avoid creasing/folding. Never store leather or suede in plastic, as moisture can build up and damage it. Have leather and suede pieces professionally dry-cleaned before they are stored. When hanging them, leave approximately two inches on either side to allow air circulation and to prevent crushing. Remember, leather is skin, so it is very sensitive to extremes in heat and cold, sunlight, and moisture.

storing

fur coats

Kim Akhtar, owner of Garde Robe in New York City, has cold storage on the premises so that clients' furs can be ready for an unforeseen trip or unexpected event. Most professional furriers do have a cold storage vault either on- or off-site. If you keep your fur coat in your own closet or basement, even if it's air-conditioned during the summer, it will dry out and the humidity will damage the quality of the fur.

Here are some of her professional tips for choosing a storage facility:

* If at all possible, ask to be shown the storage space. Make sure that no light is allowed to enter the vault.
* Make sure that the company doesn't use mothballs or sachets of any kind, as fur absorbs smells.
* The storage vault should have good air circulation and be kept at a temperature between 45 and 50 degrees Fahrenheit (7 to 10 degrees Celsius) with a humidity of 50 percent. Ask about this.
* Check the company's insurance policy and find out if your coat is covered by your homeowner's policy.
* Always have the facility where your coat is being stored check the pockets to make sure they are clean and free of dust or dirt, as this could dry out your fur.
* Storage costs vary depending on where you store your coat. In New York City, the price ranges from $90 to $300 for the season.

SHOP YOUR CLOSET

Now the closets are clean, the shopping is complete, and the unwanted clothing has been donated, consigned, or thrown away. It's time to get that closet ready for your wardrobe. Let's start by exploring the logistics of closet organization and discover what you'll need to buy and how to actually put these things to use—from shelves to bins, hangers to hooks—to make your closet a space that will enhance your life on a daily basis. Don't be frightened; you don't have to be Mr. or Ms. Fix-It to get this accomplished. Turn to chapter 4, "Rack 'Em and Stack 'Em: Implementing Your Personal Closet System," to begin.

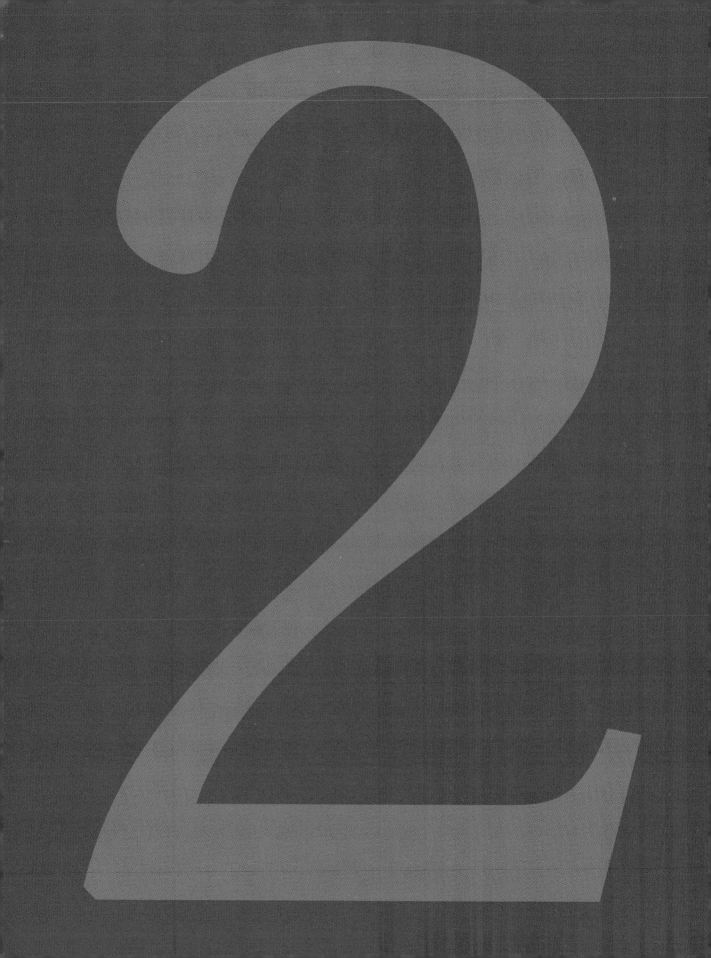

IN THE CLOSET

How many times have you looked at that toppling pile of sweaters, those squished hanging silk blouses, those boots shoved in the dark recesses of your closet and thought, *There's got to be a better way to store this stuff*? Or if you have taken the initiative and installed shelves, bins, or racks, how often have you considered the money and time spent putting in these storage saviors but acknowledged that they just aren't working? In this section of *Shop Your Closet*, we get down to the nitty-gritty, the nuts and realized bolts, so to speak, of fitting out your closet. Just when you thought you didn't have enough space, that your closet setup was hopeless, we'll show you how to effectively use the existing space and create additional space that you didn't know existed. First, we'll help you determine what type of closet you have—walk-in, reach-in, or wardrobe— and how best to outfit that closet to provide you with maximum efficiency and storage options. Then, we'll explain how to deal with the logistics of closet organization and help you discover what tools to buy and how to make those products—from hangers to hooks—work for you every day. Say good-bye to piles of wrinkled clothes, tangles of hangers, heaps of shoes and accessories, and a disorganized closet that you can't use. Turn the page and discover what you can do to end this dilemma once and for all.

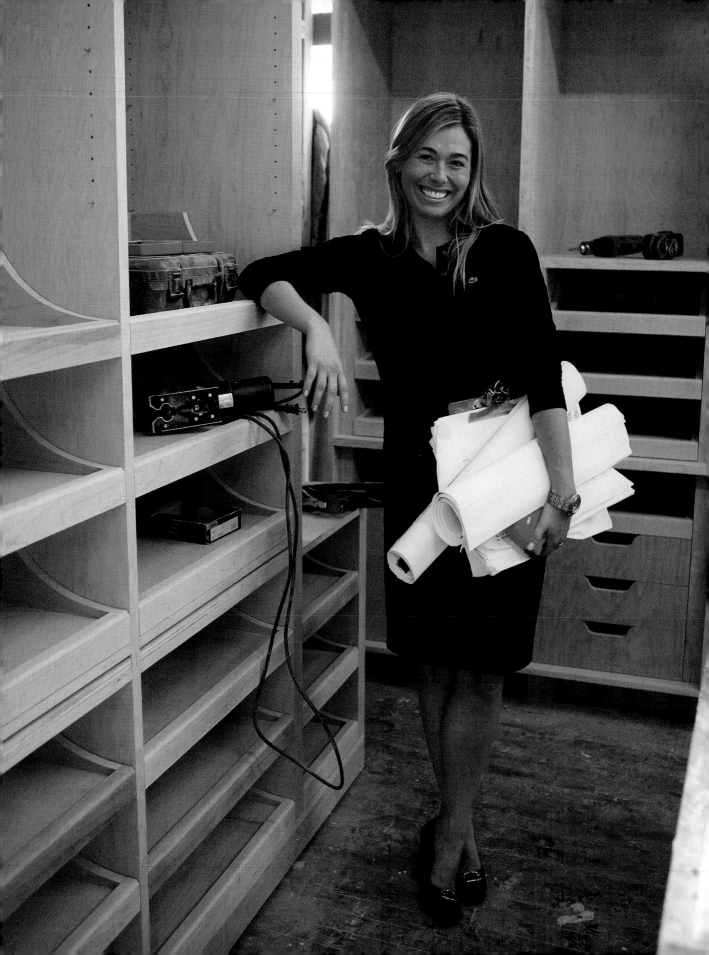

CHAPTER 4

Rack 'Em and Stack 'Em: Implementing Your Personal Closet System

FIRST THINGS FIRST—MEASURE AND TEST

Installing shelves may seem like *Mission: Impossible* to some of us, but it doesn't have to be so difficult. I know that when I was a kid, I would add shelves and bins as my wardrobe changed. If I could do it when I was 12, anyone can. For those of you who need new shelves—or closet rods or anything else that requires fastening to a wall—this chapter will explain easy ways to install them, without enlisting the costly services of a cabinetmaker or contractor. The first thing to do is measure the dimensions of your closet so that when you go to buy shelves or rods you'll know what size to buy. Do not use a ruler, a piece of string, or the length of your foot. Use a tape measure, and be certain to get an accurate measurement. If you're unsure of how to measure properly, ask a friend for help.

When installing anything that attaches to a wall, whether it's a hook, a closet rod, or shelves, the next step is to figure out what type of walls you have—Sheetrock (a brand of drywall), masonry, or plaster. This will determine what type of anchors or screw encasements that you need for proper installment.

Drywall? Masonry? Plaster? How am I supposed to figure out what type of walls I have, you're thinking. Relax. A simple wall test will help you solve the mystery.

To do a wall test, drill a small exploratory hole into the wall. If you don't have a drill, borrow one from a friend, and if you've never used a drill before, ask your friend or someone who knows how to use one to help you. Also, before you start drilling, choose a spot that is not easily visible. "If the drill easily penetrates a thickness of about three-quarters of an inch, then enters four to six inches of emptiness," says expert cabinetmaker Archie McAlister, "chances are that you are dealing with a Sheetrock wall. If, on the other hand, you find a lot of resistance, you have hit masonry or plaster." To differentiate between masonry and plaster, examine the dust that results from drilling, says McAlister. If the dust is red, you have brick or terracotta, which means your walls are made of masonry. If, however, the dust is white, chances are that you have plaster walls. If it's still unclear what types of walls you have, consult with your building's superintendent, a knowledgeable friend, or a contractor (if you're willing to spend the money).

Lead anchors are best for walls that are solid, such as plaster or masonry walls, while an E-Z Ancor, a brand of fastener, can be used for drywall. (An E-Z Anchor fastener is a bolt with fold-down side pieces that resemble wings. When the anchor is installed into the wall, the side pieces expand, holding it in place.) For greater resistance in walls made of heavier-duty drywall, you can also use toggle bolts. If you're not sure which one you need, check your local hardware store or home-improvement center and ask for help.

creating your perfect home fix-it kit

Whether you live in the tiniest studio apartment in the city or the grandest many-storied suburban mansion, you will need a basic tool kit to handle the small fix-it jobs around your home. You don't have to go out and buy an elaborate 400-piece tool kit with its own worktable at your local hardware store or home-improvement center. A simple plastic storage container with a handle (easy to purchase and simple to store), containing these few basic tools, will prove to be an invaluable aid for many of your simple home-improvement needs. One of the best gifts I received when I graduated from college was a simple but handy tool set from an eccentric aunt. It's been almost 10 years and I still have it and use it!

* *Hammer:* Buy one with a claw end so that you can easily remove nails.
* *Screwdrivers:* You will need a Phillips Head screwdriver (the one with the pointed cross-shaped end) and a slotted screwdriver (the type with a straight edge) to install and remove screws.
* *Drill:* Either battery-operated (cordless) or electrical, this tool is a great asset for your home fix-it kit. If you purchase a cordless model, be sure that it comes with

a recharger to save on battery costs. Also, if you purchase a drill, buy a small bit selection for it. The various size bits, or tips, will allow you to drill different size holes and will be very handy.

* *Tape measure:* Don't buy the ribbon style; buy a good contractor-style model with a self-locking mechanism. Buy one that is least 20 feet in length to allow you greater measuring flexibility.

* *Extension cord:* If you have an electric-powered drill, an extension cord is a must.

* *Flashlight:* Keeping a flashlight in your tool kit ensures that you will always have illumination when you need it for working in those dark, awkward spaces in your home (the closet, under the sink, behind large pieces of furniture). Make sure it has batteries that work!

* *Sharpened pencil with an eraser:* As simple as this seems, a sharpened pencil is one of the most necessary tools for your kit. The eraser removes stray pencil marks from walls, woodwork, and surfaces while you are working and can be used to remove smudge marks from painted surfaces. The sharp end is great for calculating measurements.

* *Level:* This wonderful and simple tool provides an accurate reading to make sure your shelves are level and your pictures straight.

* *Bandages/first-aid ointment:* A box of bandages and a tube of antibacterial/antiseptic ointment are great additions to your home fix-it kit. This way, if you get a minor scratch or cut while you're working, you know where the first-aid supplies are.

THREE DEGREES OF CLOSETRY

There are three types of basic closet: the walk-in (we like to refer to it as "the ultimate"), the reach-in, and the wardrobe. To figure out which one you have, read on.

* *The walk-in (the ultimate):*
The be-all, end-all of closets, the ultimate or walk-in closet is the object of every woman's desire: You have endless room to properly hang all your clothes (including that long Carolina Herrera evening gown), plenty of shoe space to be able to survey your shoe kingdom with one look, a separate dressing area (or vanity) where you can apply makeup and fix your hair, and a chair and ottoman to sit on and put on shoes or just relax and visually soak in your wardrobe. You may also have three-way mirrors, artwork, a safe to securely lock away your jewelry and other valuables, and perhaps a television or stereo! And, these fabulous custom closets are an enhancement to the value of your home. "Closets today are no longer an afterthought; they are rooms unto themselves and as important as any other in the house. Sometimes, a buyer will only purchase a home with great closet space, and this can make or break a deal," says Heather Woolems of Sotheby's International Realty, Palm Beach.

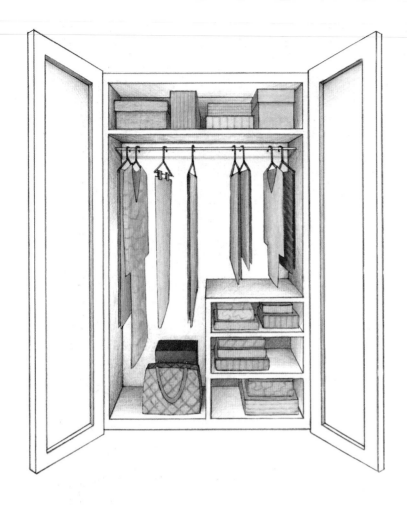

* *The reach-in:* Ranging from 72 to 96 inches deep, this is the most common species of closet. You won't be able to walk inside, but your clothes hang facing you, and you have either one long hanging bar or a long and a short hanging bar. Because of the limited storage space in most reach-in closets, it is almost more important to customize a reach-in than to customize a walk-in.

* *The wardrobe or armoire:* This freestanding cabinet can either serve as a typical reach-in closet or be customized to house shoes, handbags, or winter clothes.

A CLEAN, WELL-LIGHTED PLACE

Pulling a look together is impossible if you can't see your options, so before doing anything else, make sure you have ample light.

The Walk-In If you're lucky enough to have a walk-in, the best option is to install track lighting or overhead recessed lamps. A decorative chandelier or wall sconces can add a touch of Hollywood glamour and some ambient light as well.

The Reach-In Installing an overhead light—one with a switch or one that has a pull cord—is ideal. Battery-powered bright lights can be a good option if you're on a shoestring budget or don't have the ability to have an electrical fixture installed.

The Wardrobe The key to liking a wardrobe is to make sure that the room is well lit. If your bedroom is dim, you may want to get another lamp or two to place near the cabinet so you can easily see its contents.

CLOSET RODS

Because you'll want your hangers to glide freely along your closet rod, metal and wood are the materials of choice. If you select wood rods, keep in mind that they must be properly sanded for your hangers to slide easily. Avoid cheaply constructed closet rods, especially those made of plastic. Plastic tends to bend under the weight of clothing and will break, leaving your clothes in a huge catastrophic pile on the floor of your closet. If at all possible, fasten your closet rod directly to the wall (the flanges or the portion that attaches to the wall should be mounted using anchors appropriate for your wall type), rather than having it fit in mounts. Over time, these mounts may detach from the wall and cause the rod to slip.

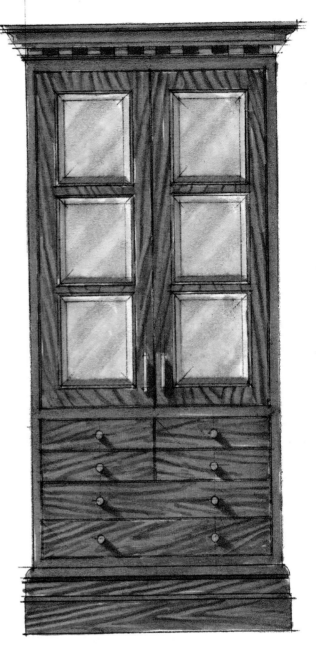

The Walk-In In the ultimate closet, make sure that your closet rods are installed horizontally on either side of the entrance, so that when you walk in, the clothing will be to your left and right. Use the back of the closet to install shelving.

The Reach-In You should maintain one reach-in with a long hanging bar, and if you have a second closet, install an additional closet rod beneath the main one.

The Wardrobe The type of rods you install will depend on what your needs are. If you are using the wardrobe to store specific items, you may have all shelves or all shoe containers or perhaps just one bar for long gowns and skirts. If the wardrobe will serve as an all-purpose closet, use a combination of these features.

TIP OF THE TRADE: Your closet must have a minimum of 84 inches in height to have room for two rods. Hang the top rod at about 81¾ inches and the lower at 40½ inches.

SHELVES

Clothes folded and placed on shelves are a lot more visible and accessible than those shoved in drawers, and having visible stacks offers a strong incentive to keep things neat! Sweaters and tees should be folded, and if you don't have room for all of your pants to be hung, perhaps fold a few pairs of jeans as well.

Shelves can be made of various materials, including wood/plywood, plastic, laminate, glass, and metal. Shelf kits are available at many home-improvement centers and organizational stores. But the easiest solution is to buy individual wood boards at your local lumberyard or hardware store.

Try to select a wood that has few knotholes or imperfections, as they can affect the stability of your shelf. Also, pick boards that are in good shape—not warped—and require as little sanding as possible. If you decide to buy plywood, make sure that it is thick enough (at least one-half inch or thicker) to be able to hold your stuff without bowing or collapsing. Plywood should be "finish grade" (good-quality wood that is ready for a simple coat of paint or stain) and won't look as if you picked it up out of your neighbor's trash or off the street on garbage night. Standard plywood sheets can be pretty rough and full of knotholes and other imperfections. To turn them into beautiful pieces of wood is simply not worth the effort. If you are unsure about what type of wood to purchase or what you will need to support the shelves, ask for help.

Shelves can be finished in either paint or stain. The choice is up to you and depends on what works best with your home's décor. If you do choose to paint your shelves, select a semigloss or gloss paint for easy maintenance. Scuff marks and dirt can be easily wiped off these paints with a damp cloth without marring the finish.

selecting the "best" shelf material

* *Wood/plywood:* This is the most common type of material used for shelves. Wood is easy to work with and can be easily trimmed to fit into any space. This extremely sturdy material can withstand a great deal of weight and can be easily finished in paint or stain to match any décor. Plywood is composed of sheets of wood that have been glued together and compressed into a solid sheet.
* *Plastic:* Plastic shelves are good choices for holding lightweight items. Their composition makes them easy to clean and they are usually sold in easy-to-assemble and easy-to-install kits at your local home-improvement store.

- *Laminate.* These extremely durable shelves are made of a core of plywood or particleboard that has had a plastic or polymer finish sheet applied to either side. Laminate shelves are easy to maintain and can support very heavy objects. However, their sturdy construction makes them extremely heavy and potentially difficult to install.
- *Glass.* Sheets of tempered glass (glass that has been manufactured to break into small pieces when shattered) is a good shelf choice if your items are going to be displayed for visual appeal. Glass shelves are not recommended for storage, as they can break easily.
- *Metal.* Metal shelves are usually sold in kits as units and are easy to put together and install. A perfect solution for storage in basements, attics, crawlspaces, and out-of-the-way places, their durability and strength make them excellent choices for storing heavy items such as large pieces of luggage, packed boxes, and sporting equipment.

The Walk-In If you have at least 12 inches of extra space above your closet rod, always add a shelf. If you have more than two and a half feet of extra space, install two shelves for additional storage space.

The Reach-In Like the walk-in, reach-ins should always have a shelf above the hanging bar. Items that should be folded, such as sweaters and tees, are best housed here. Vertical partitions or dividers should be used to help keep piles from toppling over.

The Wardrobe If you have the space and if your budget allows, you may want to consider getting a wardrobe or armoire that's loaded with shelves for your cotton knit shirts, T-shirts, and sweaters. The number of shelves that you should have in your wardrobe will vary according to its size and intended use. If you're using your wardrobe primarily to store foldable items that don't fit in your reach-in closet, you'll want the entire cabinet to be shelved. You can either purchase a ready-made wardrobe to suit your needs or customize a ready-made wardrobe (see "The Custom Wardrobe," page 69). If you're using your wardrobe as a substitute for a reach-in closet, allot space for both a hanging rod and shelving. Use your clothing inventory sheet (see the sample one on page 153) to figure out how many items need to be hung and how many need to be folded. Or if you have the space and finances available, you may want to buy two wardrobes: one for hanging and one for folding.

TIP OF THE TRADE: Shelves for folded clothing (not including sweaters) should be placed about 12 inches apart from one another, allowing for stacks that aren't unmanageably high. If you're stacking sweaters, leave 18 to 24 inches.

GETTING HOOKED

While hanging and folding takes care of most of your clothes, some things—such as robes, handbags with long shoulder straps, some belts, and jewelry accessories such as beaded necklaces—are best stored on hooks.

The most important element of hook shopping is picking out ones that work with your wall type as well as what you need them for. Hooks come in a variety of styles and can be made of plastic or metal. Hooks with large ends are great for hanging items with thick straps such as handbags, small carry-ons, and totes. Hooks with smaller ends are good for hanging belts, nightgowns and pajamas, and bathrobes. Make sure to properly anchor them, paying attention to your wall type, so that they don't come loose and fall out. If you're uncertain what style of hook is best for your specific need, ask the sales associate at your local hardware store, home-improvement center, or organizational/specialty shop for assistance.

The walk-in, the reach-in, the wardrobe—any closet can benefit from hooks. Always put at least one hooks on the back of a door to hang robes, shirts that need to go to the dry cleaner, or other things you use a lot. If you have enough space on the back wall of your closet that won't interfere with proper hanging and hanger movement, you may also want to put a few hooks here to hang winter satchels, garment bags used for travel, or other items that are seasonally or seldom used. Hanging a series of small hooks on a side wall can also be a good way to store multiple belts and scarves.

SHOE SHELVES AND RACKS

Do you find yourself buying more shoes than anything else? Are shoes the one item you can't bring yourself to edit out of your wardrobe, because stilettos rarely go out of style? Many of us suffer from shoe mania (you can include me in this illustrious group). But how do you keep all those wonderful darlings organized?

It is no secret that many fashionistas keep their footwear in boxes with a photo taped to the end so that they know which pair of stilettos lives where. But boxes are clunky and often take up more space than is needed. Shoe shelves are a more practical way to store your beloved footwear.

The Walk-In Slanted shoe shelves are ideal for women's shoes, while larger and bulkier men's shoes can be placed on flat shelves. These can be custom-built or purchased at home-improvement and home-organization stores.

The Reach-In If you have the space, it's best to have some shoe shelves on the floor of your reach-in, under the long hanging bar. If the floor shelves don't offer enough room for all of your shoes, keep your most frequently used pairs on the shelves and store your others, perhaps in clear boxes or shoe drawers, under your bed.

The Wardrobe You may want to consider customizing a shoe rack, either by inserting individual wooden shoe compartments into the wardrobe base or by hanging canvas shoe racks. Both wooden shoe compartments and hanging canvas racks can be found at home-organization stores across the country, on the Internet, and in catalogues. If you are a true shoe fanatic and have the available space, consider devoting an entire wardrobe to shoe storage!

the custom wardrobe

If you find that you've followed all the tips given to maximize space in your closet—walk-in or reach-in—but still can't store all that you own, you may want to invest in a custom wardrobe for your extras. The main incentive behind the custom wardrobe is specificity. Whether the extra space you need is for storing accessories, sweaters, shoes, pants, or your significant other's clothes, avoid the tangled mess of your pack rat days. Storing your shoes with your partner's belts is the first step toward reinstating closet chaos!

* *Multiaccessory:* Need extra space for your handbags, shoes, scarves, and belts? A wardrobe may be the perfect

solution. Buy either an empty wardrobe or one with adjustable shelving on which you can stack handbags and scarves. On the bottom shelves, insert shoe compartments that you can find at a local home goods or organization specialty store. The back of the doors (or singular door, in the case of an old-fashioned wardrobe) is a good spot to tack a row of hooks for hanging your belts. Voilà! You have a perfectly organized place to easily locate the perfect handbag, belt, and shoe combination.

* *Shoes:* Say you have 60 pairs of shoes in need of a viable storage solution. A wardrobe, outfitted with clear plastic open-ended boxes—or shoe compartments as mentioned above—can make the perfect home for your shoes!

* *Clothing:* Are you a sweater freak or a major gym rat with stacks of yoga pants, bra tops, and exercise tees? (Or a combination of both?!) Rather than jamming your closet shelves full of it all, consider purchasing a freestanding chest of drawers, a shelf unit, or an armoire to hold these stacks.

Now, some of you may say, "Wait a minute, my closet is sort of a reach-in, but it has some qualities of a wardrobe or a walk-in." These unique closet creations have problems of their own. Below are some problems and their solutions to help you. Remember, the main purpose is to adequately and safely store your clothing, while allowing you the best access to make your wardrobe as attainable and wearable as possible.

PROBLEM: *I have two parallel rods, one in front of the other in a deep closet that creates a blind corner that becomes cluttered and makes getting the things stored there hard to reach. What should I do?*

SOLUTION: This issue is fairly common in older buildings and pre–World War II apartments in urban areas, where closets were built very wide and deep. A good, fairly simple solution is to add a bin to that corner so that you can pull out the entire contents in an orderly manner, get what you need, then return it to its place.

PROBLEM: *I have a closet with a very high ceiling. How can I best use that dead space?*

SOLUTION: The best way to maximize this valuable space for storage is to install clear or acrylic shelves. This will allow you to see what you have stored in that area, without creating a black hole.

PROBLEM: *I have no room for a mirror in my room, and I really need one when I get dressed. What can I do?*

SOLUTION: Put a full-length mirror on the back of your closet door. This is the simplest answer to this conundrum. And, if you have the space and the money, a decadent solution is to install a three-panel mirror, with fabric on the back of the two side panels. When the two side panels are folded in, they can double as an inspiration board or a place to pin and display your jewelry.

Now that you have your closet decked out with all the storage enhancements you need, you may ask yourself: *What do I hang? What do I fold?* Read the next chapter—"To Hang and to Fold"—to give yourself a better idea of how to best store your wardrobe.

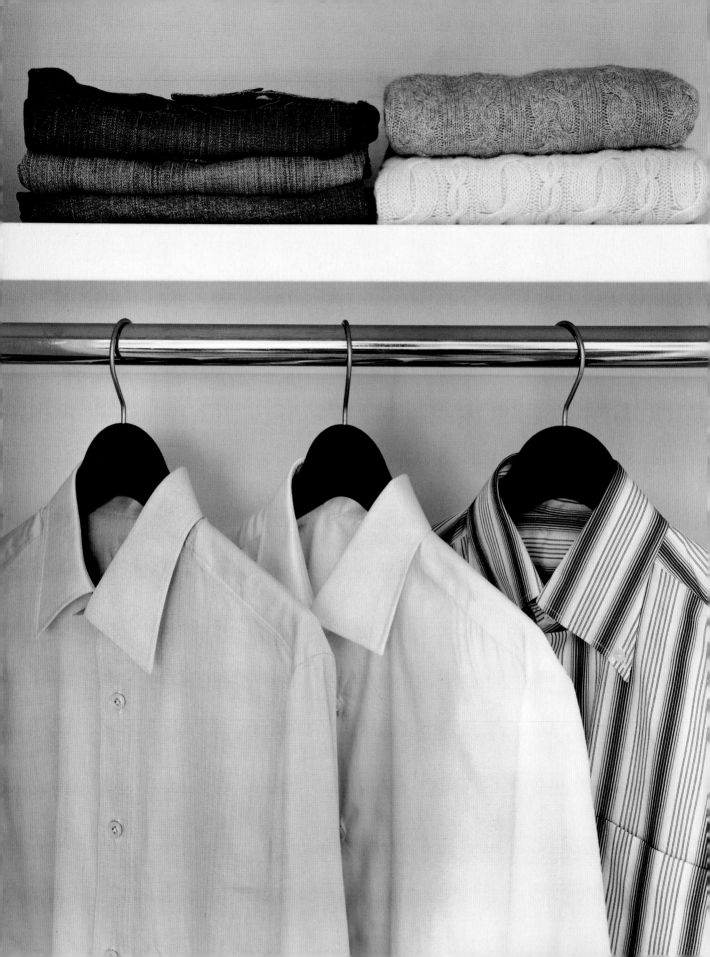

CHAPTER 5

To Hang and to Fold

You've edited your wardrobe, donated or consigned your unwanted clothing, thrown out the stuff that was too damaged or stained to give away, and installed shelves, rods, hooks, and other necessary organizational accoutrements to make your closet the envy of the neighborhood and an organizational dream. Now you are ready for the next step—putting your clothes away. Great. But do you hang it or fold it? And how do you hang it and fold it? This next critical step will prevent the death and destruction of your beloved clothing. You don't want your $500 suede skirt ruined with a permanent crease or your beautiful raspberry cashmere sweater stretched out of shape by being hung on a (gasp!) wire hanger. Read on to get the answers you seek.

TO HANG OR TO FOLD?
THAT IS THE QUESTION

Don't panic. The hang-versus-fold conundrum is easier to solve than you think. Certain pieces absolutely, positively, undoubtedly and always must be hung—coats, pants, dresses, suits, tailored shirts, silk blouses, gowns, and any article of clothing that is too bulky or too awkward to be folded or requires that its shape is best kept by being placed on a hanger. And when things are stored on hangers, it's easier to see what the item is and easier to shop your closet (hence, the title of this book). However, some things are destined to be folded—sweaters, underwear/lingerie, sport/gym clothing, T-shirts, socks, delicate clothing (beaded apparel, lace garments, cashmere, and fine knits) and jeans (if you don't have the space to hang them!). These things can be folded and placed in bins, in drawers, on shelves, or, if space is at a major premium, stored in containers under the bed or even suitcases (this is an excellent way to deal with seasonal clothes). Hung clothing takes up less space and organizes your pieces to make using your wardrobe easier and more efficient. Not to mention it keeps your clothes looking fresher and prevents things from getting wrinkled or damaged from improper storage.

THE TEN COMMANDMENTS OF HANGING

I. *Thou shalt hang as much as possible in thy closet.* If you can hang it, you should, unless of course it's the frequently worn pair of corduroys for your two-year-old toddler, your sexy silk-and-lace nightie, or your fabulous red cashmere cowl neck. Clothing retains its shape better and is likely to look better and last longer if it is properly hung. But as with all rules, there are always exceptions—never hang delicates, such as beaded items or fine cashmere, because hanging may pull them out of shape and cause damage to the garment. Instead, fold them and place acid-free tissue around the items to help protect them.

2. *Thou shalt not hang sweaters.* Sweaters are best folded and stored on shelves or in drawers to maintain their shape.

3. *Thou shalt banish wire hangers from thy closet.* In the immortal words of Joan Crawford in *Mommie Dearest*: "No wire hangers!" Wood is ideal, plastic is fine, but those skinny, tangle-inducing wire hangers that the dry cleaners give away have got to go! They lose their shape, leave marks on your clothing, and are simply not strong enough to support the weight of any garment properly. They are a nightmare and must be banished from your life . . . forever!

4. *Thou shalt have matching hangers.* A hodgepodge of different hangers made from varying materials will make your closet look sloppy and prevent your clothes from hanging properly. The tangled, jumbled mess cramps anyone's style and pulls your eye away from the clothing. Buy hangers made from the same material. You'll be glad you did. "Having the same style hanger helps everything looks uniform and allows all your clothing to hang in the same manner," says Emilia Fanjul Pfeifler, president of EF Communications.

5. *Thou shalt use appropriate hangers for appropriate garments.* What does this mean? Simple. Hanging a coat? Use a coat hanger. The

appropriate style of the hanger will keep your coat in tip-top shape. Hanging a skirt? Use a skirt hanger. The clamps will hold the waistband of the garment securely and make it as wrinkle-free as possible.

6. *Thou shalt not kill clothes with plastic.* Those dry-cleaning bags that are lovingly placed over your garments at the cleaners are used to prevent the items from getting dirty in transit. Once those garments are securely within the confines of your home, remove the dry-cleaning plastic and throw it away. Dry-cleaning plastic can trap moisture, which can lead to bacteria and mildew/mold growth, which in turn can severely damage, discolor, or stain your clothing. Also, natural fibers such as cotton, wool, silk, and linen need to breathe. They need to have air circulating around them. So dump the plastic and make your clothes happy.

7. *Honor the breathing room of thy clothing.* While you want to hang as much as possible, leave enough space between each garment so that they're not crammed together in your closet. Cramming causes wrinkling and makes you look like you slept in your best suit. No one wants to wear a shirt that has been so tightly jammed into a closet that its neighbor's shape is imprinted on its back. If you leave adequate space, it will keep your garments looking neater and pressed and help you better see what you have to wear.

8. *Thou shalt not hang thy clothes with strangers.* Put like with like. In other words, hang shirts with shirts, pants with pants, suits with suits, and so on. And, most important, always hang clothes facing in the same direction. This way, you will be able to see and find

SHOP YOUR CLOSET

things more easily. If you have an entire outfit that you frequently wear, why not hang the pieces together? This will save time and make shopping your closet easier.

9. *Thou shalt color-code.* Organizing your clothes by color allows you to visualize an outfit by separates and helps you to mix and match combinations you might otherwise miss.

10. *Honor thy pants and thy sweaters.* Keep pants looking freshly pressed by hanging them along their creases or pleats to keep them sharp; always fold sweaters so that they don't lose their shape.

THE ANATOMY OF A HANGER

To properly hang your clothes in your closet, you'll need to learn the anatomy of a hanger. Simply put, there are specific hangers that hang certain pieces of clothing in a proper way to ensure their safe storage and to maximize their appearance when you wear them. No one wants to wear a dress with distorted shoulders or a pair of pants with lines in the wrong places. If you always use the right hanger, your clothes will always be hung properly and you'll always look your best.

The Classic

The classic hanger is multipurpose, is great for hanging shirts and jackets. Made of plastic or wood, its rigid form makes it perfect for holding heavy items such as wool pants.

All-Purpose

The all-purpose hanger sports a pair of clips that will allow you to hang pants or skirts from the clips (which must be padded to prevent them from marking your clothes) to keep their shape and press. Pants should be hung by the cuffs with the waistband facing the floor and folded on the crease; skirts should be hung by the waistband. Coordinating pairs can be hung with the jackets, blouses, tops, or vests on the main part of the hanger on top and the matching pants or skirt below. This will keep ensembles together and allow you to put on outfits that have been prematched.

The Notched

A hanger with notches cut into it prevents shoulder straps from slipping off. You can use it for dresses, silk blouses, and anything that hangs from a thin strap.

The Wide-Shoulder

The wide-shoulder hanger is best suited for heavy coats and suit jackets. The spread of the hanger helps maintain the shape of the garment and prevents the shoulders from getting out of alignment or misshapen.

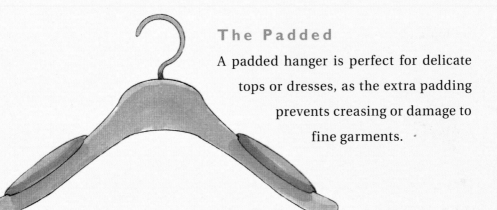

The Padded

A padded hanger is perfect for delicate tops or dresses, as the extra padding prevents creasing or damage to fine garments.

TIP OF THE TRADE: To have your hangers slide effortlessly on your closet rod, simply gently rub the entire length of the rod with a bar of soap. Don't put too much on (nobody wants soap flakes falling on their clothes!). Your hangers will glide smoothly and freely. You can also use some butcher's wax or the end of a candle to achieve the same result.

above and beyond: 11 extras that can change your life for the better

Shoe racks, shelves, and hangers aside, some other closet accessories are not imperative but will make your sartorial existence a million times better than you would have ever imagined:

* *Shoe shiners:* There are few items next to the cash register that we actually should buy when we check out—shoe shiners are one of them. These little plastic applicators have a sponge end that is infused with shoe polish for a quick fix. It's best to buy a neutral one that suits all colors and tones of shoes.

* *Bed lifts: attention, New Yorkers. . . .* And anyone else who needs more storage space than the regular under-bed space provides. Bed lifts—small plastic or metal lifts to be placed under the legs of your bed frame—are a cheap and easy way to provide an extra 6 to 15 inches of space for bigger containers to hold bulky sweaters, linens, and extra drapes or towels.

* *Lavender sweater folds:* Bought in specialty stores, lavender sweater folds are essentially good smelling bean bags that help your wooly knits, cables, and cashmeres stay in good shape. A natural antiseptic, lavender also helps keep the bugs at bay.

* *Professional or portable steamer:* Save yourself hours of ironing with the flick of a switch. Professional steamers vary in price, but most average about $100, not exactly cheap. So if you'd rather spend your cash elsewhere, buy a portable one that costs about $25. Note that portable steamers are not quite as powerful, but they can be easily stored and are great for travel.

SHOP YOUR CLOSET

* *Lint removers:* An absolute must for anyone! The best thing about these invaluable wardrobe enhancers is that you can buy them at your local drugstore, supermarket, or variety store for about $1.99.

* *Dividers.* Dividers are one of the great unsung heroes of organizational products. Made of plastic, wood, or acid-free cardboard, these organizational godsends come in a variety of heights and depths for different sizes of your shelves. (Think of them as bookends for your closet.) Those without them may think they're ridiculous, but how else are you supposed to keep your stack of sweaters from toppling over?

* *Drawer organizers.* Underwear and socks are best kept in drawers, and—let's be honest—no one wants to spend valuable time trying to fold a thong. Drawer organizers make a section for separate undergarments the way a fishing tackle box separates one lure from another.

* *Felt-lined jewelry trays:* Whether you have splashy costume baubles or exquisite five-carat diamonds, setting a drawer aside for your jewels will make getting dressed up all the easier. And felt jewelry trays—preferably the kind that stack one on top of the other— will help you keep your necklaces, bracelets, and earrings free of scratches and tangles.

* *Stepladder/step stool:* How can you expect yourself to wear your sweaters if they're stacked way out of your reach? Stepladders are an inexpensive way to make sure you use that extra space, not only in your closets but also in

your kitchen! And they are the proper way to reach those out-of-the-way places in your closet. Do not stand on a chair, a box, or a stack of books—you risk falling and injuring yourself.

* *A junk trunk:* No matter how much de-pack-rat-ifying we do, we'll still be stuck with replacement buttons, safety pins, receipts for potential returns, and other items that need housing. Invest in a small box or miniature chest of drawers where you can keep these items. This way, the next time that button falls off your winter coat, you'll know where to find the replacement.

* *Folding board:* Folding your sweaters and shirts uniformly will make your stacks look better and help save space. Invest in a folding board at your local organizational store. Or cut a 10-inch by 12-inch piece of durable cardboard to create a homemade folding board.

KNOW WHEN TO FOLD 'EM

It's hard sometimes to decide whether to hang them or fold clothing. Hanging, as we talked about earlier, is preferable to folding because it allows for your clothes to be more economically stored and helps you truly see what you have in your closet. But as we also noted, some things—

82 SHOP YOUR CLOSET

sweaters, underwear, sporting clothes, delicates (beaded items and cashmere)—are best folded.

To neatly and uniformly fold your clothing, use a folding board that can be purchased at an organizational or home-furnishings store. Or you can make your own homemade version by cutting a 10-inch by 12-inch piece of durable cardboard. Make certain the cuts are even and that there are no sharp edges. This simple item will make folding a snap and will create uniform stacks that will look better and conserve space in your closet.

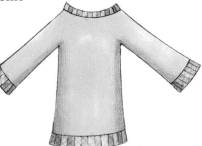

When folding sweaters, use lavender sweater folds (basically, beanbags filled with lavender, which smells wonderful) to help all your sweaters, from cashmeres and cable-knits to wooly ski sweaters and angora turtlenecks, maintain their shape. The weight of the bag helps keep the shape of your folded item and the added bonus of the lavender (a natural antiseptic) will keep the bugs at bay, leaving your sweaters hole-free and smelling as fresh as a morning in the south of France!

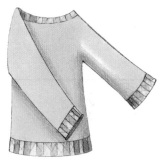

When placing your folded treasures on your shelves, remember to keep the stacks neat and use dividers (available at organizational and home-furnishing stores) to maintain their upright position. Nobody wants to open up their closet and see little leaning towers of Pisa. Dividers are also a great way to separate your socks and underwear in a drawer or bin.

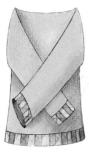

You've hung, you've folded, and your closet is looking great! Turn to chapter 6 to discover the art of handling your precious accessories.

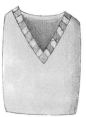

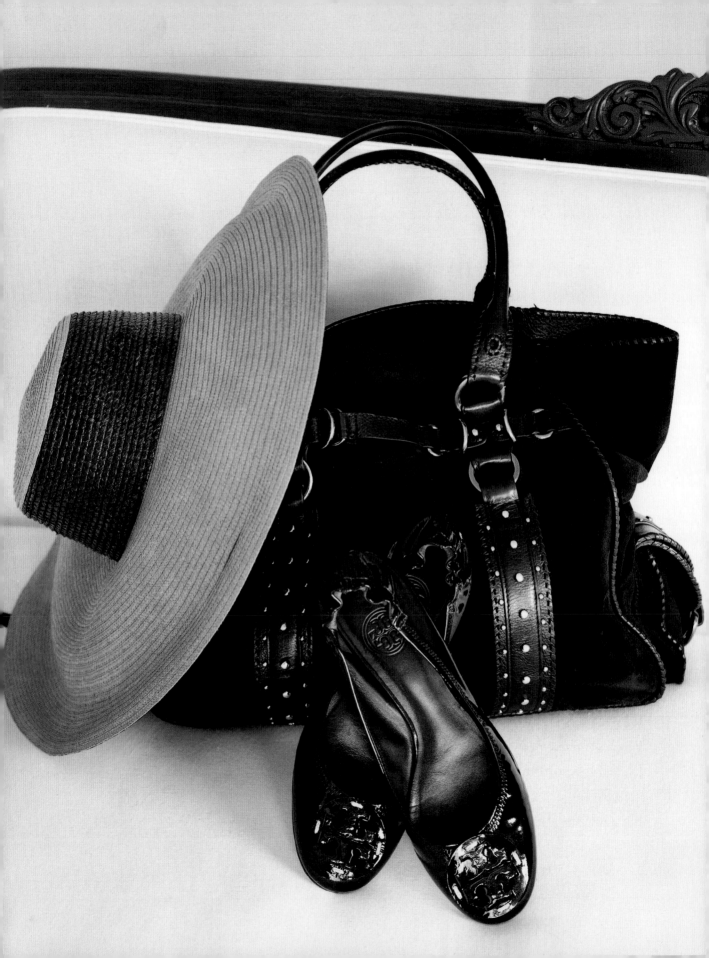

Handling Handbags, Shoes, Scarves, Belts, and Jewelry

Since childhood, I have had a fascination with organization and closet design. We moved a lot, and when my parents were having their first custom home built, my dad allowed me free reign over my bedroom; I was 10 and he was letting me design my own closet. It was heaven! When I was finished, I am proud to say my closet was the be-all and end-all; there was a place for everything, from my favorite party dresses to my vast collection of gym clothes and school uniforms. But it was my clever design solutions for my accessories that blew them away. I had special trays and little dividers in drawers to display and store my "jewelry," an amazing hook system to hold my purses and book bags, and an ingenious storage nook for my suitcases and sports equipment. Even my shoes had their own special rack! My parents were so amazed and impressed that I was put in charge of closet design for the entire house. My mom's costume jewelry collection was organized to the nth degree with all types of jewelry dividers in the drawers, and my dad's ties were the picture of perfection, organized by color and style.

THE FINISHING TOUCH: ACCESSORIES

Great shoes, a fantastic handbag, an elegant scarf, a statement-making belt, or a drop-dead piece of jewelry, pinned to your lapel, can transform an ensemble from drab to fab, so proper care and visible storage with easy access is key for these vital fashion finishing touches. Don't let these important details flounder in the bottom of your closet in an undistinguishable heap. Rescue your accessories from their illicit hiding places in your home and give them their proper place of prominence within your closet.

Handbag Heaven

Handbags, the all-important wardrobe essential, demand respect. They are your personal valet, your constant companion that cares for and carries all of life's important stuff—keys, wallet, money, identification, important papers, tissues, eyeglasses, medication, lipstick, comb, and whatever else you need to carry with you through the day. Most of us have many different handbags in assorted materials and colors to match various outfits and to coordinate with the seasons. But be honest. How do you store your handbags when you are not using them—in a pile on the floor of your closet? Hanging on the various doorknobs throughout your home? Slung over the posts on your headboard or footboard? Thrown underneath your bed? This simply won't do.

The best way to store handbags is to hang them from S-shaped hooks on a rod in your closet or lined up on a shelf. Be careful not to hang them too close together, or they may get damaged or entangled. Also, as with the rest of your wardrobe, separate them by color and style. This way, if you are looking for a particular style of handbag, it will be easier to locate what you want without having to look through your entire collection.

Empty Your Bag, Lady

Never store handbags full of stuff. Not only will doing so make it difficult for you to remember where you have your passport and check-book stashed, but also, handbags crammed full of life's flotsam and jet-sam will lose their shape and become damaged. When you're going to store a handbag, empty its con-tents. Throw away any unneces-sary pieces of paper, old lipstick tubes, and loose mints and put away your wallet, keys, eyeglasses, passport, checkbook, and other essentials in a location where you can easily find them and transfer them to your new handbag. Stuff the inside of the bag with acid-free tissue. Do not overstuff. (You don't want your handbags to resemble a row of Thanksgiving turkeys about ready to burst their seams!) As with shoes, check them for scuffs, scratches, and nicks. If your bag is leather, polish it. If you don't know what color polish to get, buy one in a neutral shade. This way, any scuffs or scratches will be removed and the color will not be affected. If your bag is suede, brush it with a suede brush, making sure to keep the nap going in one direction. Do not use a toothbrush, hairbrush, or any other brush that is not meant to be used on suede. If your bag has a scratch or spot and you have no idea how to get rid of it, take it to your favorite shoe-repair store or ask your local dry cleaner for advice. Sometimes a store or boutique where you purchase your handbags is a good source for tips on care. Or you can try to contact the manufacturer via the Internet or by calling. But no matter what you do, never put water or any type of cleaning solution or stain-removal product on your handbag without checking with the pros first.

FOR THE LOVE OF SHOES

Who could ever forget Carrie on *Sex and the City* and her vast collection of shoes? For many of us, shoes are the holy grail of fashion shopping. Names such as Manolo Blahnik, Jimmy Choo, and Prada can bring many of us to our knees!

Like other accessories, a phenomenal pair of shoes can transform your all-purpose little black dress into a cocktail-party knockout! So as you do with those handbags, treat these babies with respect and care, and they will give you years of pleasure and panache.

Storing Shoes

There are three basic ways to best store your shoes: in pairs on a flat shelf, in pairs on a slanted shelf, or in open-ended shoe boxes that can be stacked. Whatever you choose, on the basis of space, personal preference, or ease, remember that before you do any storing, your shoes must be in the best possible condition. Special forms called shoe trees are available at your local organization store, home-furnishings boutique, specialty shop, or chain store, such as Target, Linens 'n Things, and Bed Bath & Beyond. They are made of metal, wood, or plastic and are designed to slip inside your shoes to keep their shape. Boot trees or shapers are also available and can be used to keep your boots in their best shape. If you cannot find trees or shapers that work for your shoes, acid-free tissue is a good substitute for helping your footwear maintain its shape.

If your shoes have mud or other debris on them, brush them off and polish if needed. Check your laces to make sure they're not rotting and full of knots. If they're in bad shape, replace them. If the soles are worn or if the taps (the protective shield placed on the heel) are missing, have new ones put on. Use your local shoe-repair shop to handle this work. Also, in many areas, dry cleaners also provide this service. If you don't know where to get your shoes repaired, check with your neighbors and coworkers and friends, look through the phone directory, or check on the Internet. A good shoe repair specialist is worth his or her weight in gold! Finally, never put away wet shoes. They invite mold or mildew and can be permanently ruined. If you're caught in a rainstorm with your favorite pair of shoes, take them off as soon as possible. Dry them carefully with a clean towel and stuff the toes with acid-free tissue or place shoe trees in them. Then, put them on top of a clean towel in a warm, well-ventilated area. Never put wet shoes on top of or too near a heat source such as a radiator or baseboard heat—the extreme heat can cause the leather to crack or buckle.

caring for leather, suede, and canvas

* *Leather:* The best way to care for leather goods such as handbags, belts, and shoes is to treat them with mink oil to help them retain their moisture. Think of it as a moisturizer for the things you wear. To help them keep their shine, use a neutral shoe polish or a shoe shiner (a plastic applicator loaded with a neutral polish available at drugstores, supermarkets, and chain stores) daily. After applying the polish, let it dry and buff the shoes to shine with a clean cloth. If your shoes are scratched or scuffed, use a tinted shoe polish in a color that matches the color of your shoes. If your shoes are an unusual color or if the scratch is fairly deep, take them to your local shoe-repair shop and have them professionally taken care of.

* *Suede:* To clean and maintain your favorite suede shoes, belts, and bags, use a suede brush to remove dirt and dust and to keep the nap of your item in good shape. Suede spots easily, so try to avoid wearing suede items when the weather is inclement. If you get a spot or stain on your favorite suede fashion accessory, purchase a suede cleaner. If you use them, please read the directions carefully and follow them to the letter. The best-case scenario is to take these items to your local shoe-repair shop for professional attention.

* *Canvas:* For canvas items, many times a vigorous brushing with a shoe brush will remove any smudges or light dirt. If your canvas belt, handbag, or shoes are really dirty, check to see if there is a manufacturer's tag attached to the item recommending how to clean it. Some things can be laundered (such as your favorite tennis shoes or your beach tote), but when in doubt, take the item to your local dry cleaner and ask a professional how to proceed.

TIE ONE ON—THE ART OF STORING SCARVES, BELTS, AND TIES

Scarves, ties, and belts: these elegant accessories provide a splash of color for our outfits and state who we are and how we feel. (Remember the "power tie" of the 1980s? By the way, the color was yellow, in case you forgot.) To properly store scarves, set them flat, fold them in fours, and wrap them in acid-free tissue. This will help them avoid wrinkling and keep them fresh and ready to wear. Men's ties can be stored on a tie rack. There are many styles available in the marketplace. Choose one that suits your budget and space restrictions and that can accommodate the number of pieces in your tie collection. Try to avoid folding ties, as they can become creased and lose their shape. Never leave your ties stuffed into your briefcase or coat pocket. If you get a spot or stain on your tie or scarf, take it to your favorite dry cleaner and have it professionally cleaned.

Depending on its style, a belt can be either hung on a hook or special belt hanger or, if it has a face, rolled and placed on a shelf. Like shoes and handbags, leather belts should be polished; suede belts should be brushed. Fancy belts with elaborate buckles and jewel-encrusted bands should be stored the way you would a very large piece of jewelry to avoid damage to the stones and adornments, in a separate velvet-lined box or in an individual pouch or bag made out of felt or velvet. If a specific belt is part of a coat or outfit, it should be hung with it, if at all possible, to avoid losing it.

THE FAMILY JEWELS

Most people, when they think of storing jewelry, imagine a large fancy box on top of their dresser or a bunch of little boxes stuffed into a drawer. I am not a fan of jewelry boxes for two reasons—first, they clutter up the sur-

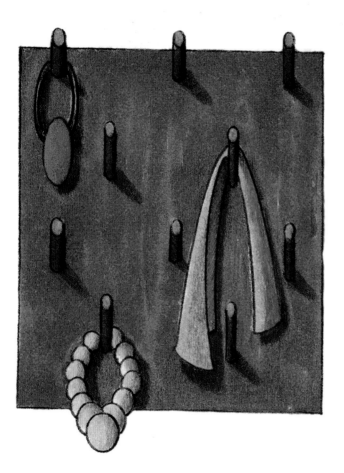

faces in your bedroom, and second, they keep your jewelry in jumbled heaps that are almost always impossible to sort. But a great way to store your jewelry, which is my favorite, is to install a pegboard in your closet. By simply inserting little hooks into the pegboard, you can sort and store your jewelry safely and easily. The pegboard allows you to easily view your pieces and prevents them from becoming entangled.

Another way to safely and easily store your favorite jewelry pieces is to buy jewelry inserts that, placed on a shelf or in a cubby, can segregate your pins from your necklaces and your bracelets from your ear-

rings. These inserts are usually lined with a soft fabric such as felt or velvet, which prevents the individual pieces from getting scratched or nicked while they are being stored.

Finally, the ultimate in attainable luxury is to have a safe installed in your closet. Although it might seem extravagant, a good safe can help protect your fine jewelry, valuables, small heirlooms, and important papers from fire and theft. And if you keep them securely stored in this ultimate storage place, you never have to wonder where you stashed them away or hid them in your home.

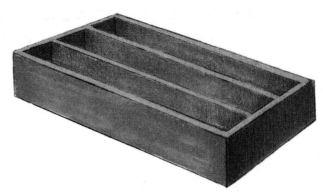

Now that we have our accessories stored, shipshape and gorgeous, we're ready to tackle the next chapter and organize those special closets in our homes—the linen closet, the coat closet, and for those of us who are privileged to have them, the kids closets.

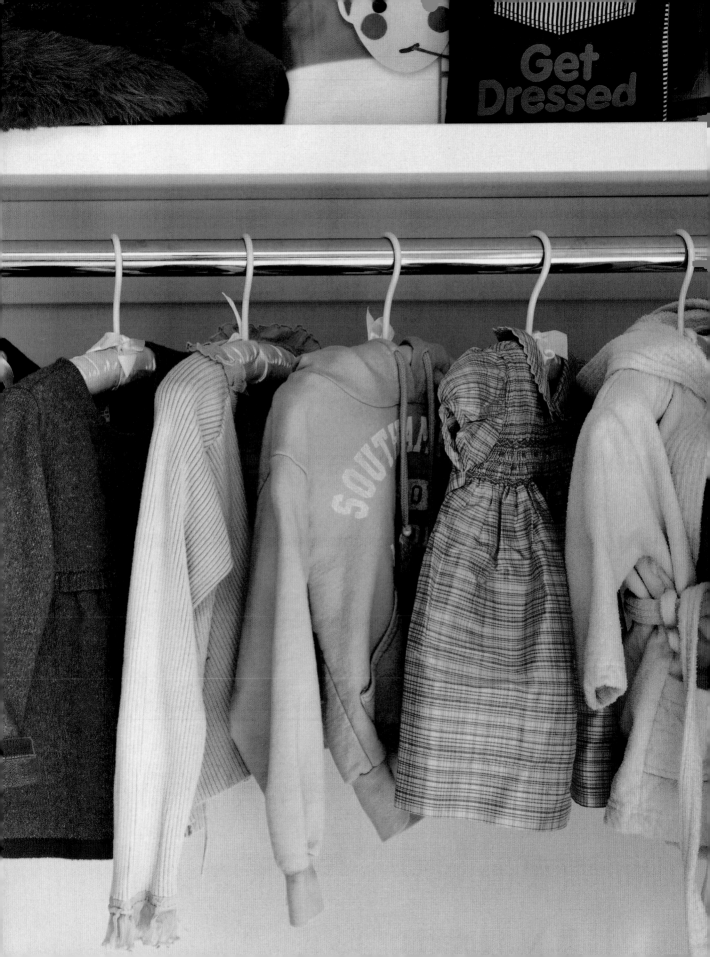

CHAPTER 7

Specialty Closets— Linen, Coats, and Kids

Your closets are looking great. Now it's time to tackle those specialty closets that most of us tend to overlook—linen, coats, and kids. How many times have you gone into the linen closet for a clean towel only to find a jumbled mess of sheets, towels, blankets, and comforters? Or how often have you looked for your child's left shoe and spent an unseemly amount of time rummaging through toys, games, books, clothing, and goodness knows what else in the bottom of his closet? When company comes over and you try to hang your visitors' coats in the coat closet, do you find it stuffed with clothes, sporting equipment, umbrellas, and an odd assortment of the stuff that seems to endlessly accumulate? Read on to transform these specialty closets from cluttered chaos into spectacular storage.

THE LINEN CLOSET

Unlike most other closets, the linen closet, that special place in your home where you store all your towels, sheets, pillowcases, facecloths, blankets, tablecloths, napkins, and so on, is unusual in that all of its contents are folded and not hung. The secret of keeping this closet tidy and organized is simple: efficient and neat folding to maximize space and allow you easy viewing of your household linens. This closet should contain a row of shelves designed to store your household linens—sheets (both fitted and flat), pillowcases, towels, facecloths, extra blankets and bedding, and table linens, if room allows—in tidy, folded piles. Segregate the type of linen by shelf. In other words, put all towels on the same shelf and bed linens on another one. This will make it easy for you to find fresh linens whenever you need them. When storing bed linens, try to keep complete sets together. Place the folded fitted sheet and pillowcases inside the flat sheet and fold this over the others to create a complete set. Nothing is more frustrating than mixing your twin sheets for your guest bedroom with your queen-size sheets for your bedroom. If you keep bed sheet sets together, it will cut down on the amount of time spent looking for the right pillowcases and sheets to make your bed.

folding
fitted
sheets

Folding fitted sheets can drive the sanest of us into a state of sheer rage and frustration; those weird pleated corners and the funny elastic defy reason. But if these necessities are not folded properly, the result is a horrible balled-up mess that does not sit neatly on your shelf in the linen closet and looks wrinkled and sloppy when it is finally used on the bed. Here's how to avoid that disaster:

* *Step 1:* To get the best fold possible, lay the fitted sheet on a large flat surface such as a table or bed. Place the sheet facedown, with the elastic corners facing up. Turn in the edges and corners to make a straight edge. Fold the sheet in half vertically and tuck the right top corner into the bottom right corner. Do the same for the left side. Now the sheet should be folded in half horizontally. At each corner, place your hand in each fold and smooth and flatten.
* *Step 2:* Fold the sheet in half lengthwise. Smooth the edges out.
* *Step 3:* Fold the sheet lengthwise again (reducing the width by half). Then, fold the sheet into thirds. It is now ready to be stored neatly on your shelf.

Each bed in your home should have three sets of sheets—one on the bed, one in the laundry to be washed, and one spare in the closet. Likewise, it is good to have two complete sets of towels for each person in your home. The average towel set should consist of a bath towel, a hand towel, and a facecloth. Large bath towels can also be included in the set if you like them. (These oversized towels are an attainable luxury!) Like bed sheets, bath linens should be stored in sets. This way, it's easy to see what pieces you have without searching through piles within the closet.

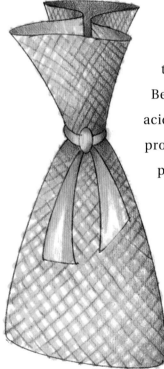

Store blankets and extra bedding such as duvet covers, comforters, and quilts in neat stacks on hard-to-reach upper shelves or at the bottom of the closet. Before storing, clean this bedding and then wrap it in acid-free tissue or in old (but clean) unused flat sheets to protect them from dirt and dust. Never store any linens in plastic, as mold or mildew can easily flourish, and for the same reason, never put freshly laundered linens away wet or damp. Make sure that these items are completely dry before putting them away, to prevent damage and staining. Nothing is more disturbing than slipping into a bed made with mildew-laden sheets or drying off after a refreshing shower with stinky towels.

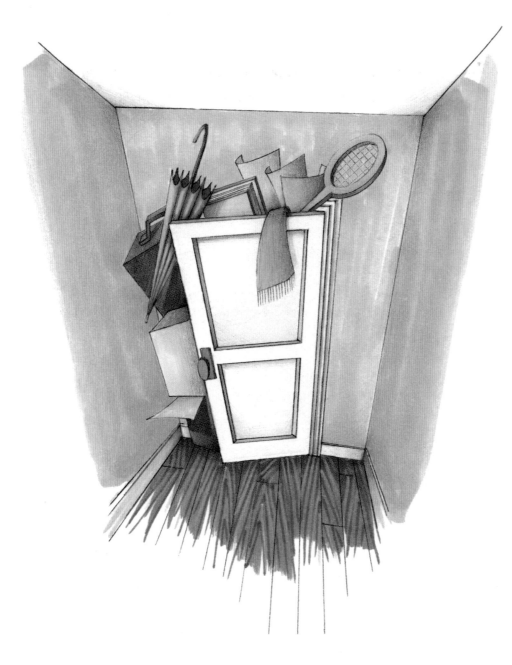

THE COAT CLOSET

You know the one. It's the closet located in your entry hall or near the front of your home that seems to be the logical place to put everything you don't have a place for—umbrellas, seasonal clothing, sporting equipment, suitcases, boxes of important papers, your college textbooks, and goodness knows what else that has found a resting spot in this domestic black hole.

If you need to get out your winter coat or ski parka or, if you're feeling particularly brave, try to hang up a visitor's coat, you cross your fingers and pray that the junk avalanche doesn't explode into the room.

The Three C's

Cool, clean, controlled—These are the secrets for safe and successful coat storage.

* *Cool* : Never store coats in an overheated or excessively hot closet, as heat can damage them. Don't forget, as discussed earlier in this book, furs should be stored in cold storage at your favorite furrier or your local dry cleaner.

* *Clean:* A clean coat closet is a happy coat closet. Make sure that the closet is dry, to avoid damaging mold and mildew and insect infestation, and dust and vacuum the closet regularly to get rid of the dust mites and dirt that can soil your coats. When storing your coats, empty the pockets beforehand, put them away after dry-cleaning, and remove the plastic from the cleaners. Some coats, such as cashmere or wool, can be stored in cloth garment bags to keep them clean and to prevent fading. Avoid mothballs, which can be dangerous if you have inquisitive children or pets, and they have a pungent smell that's hard to air out of your favorite coat. Have you ever noticed on the first cold day of the year there's always the telltale smell of mothballs lingering in a crowded subway car or on the bus or train? Instead, use lavender sachets to keep the bugs at bay and your coats smelling fresh. Cedar shavings, blocks, or balls can also be used, but you may end up smelling like a hamster cage when you slip on your winter coat.

* *Controlled:* Try to use your coat closet's hanging space only for storing your coats. Resist the urge to jam it up with extra bedding, camping gear, and boxes of your college textbooks. Keep similar styles of coats together and hang your coats on sturdy hangers all of the same material. This uniformity will ensure that your coats are hung properly and will retain their shape. Never jam your coats into the closet, as they can become entangled and cause creasing or rumpling that will make your coat look as if you slept in it. If your coat closet allows, use the shelf space above for storing suitcases and traveling bags. When storing suitcases, always put them away clean. If using them to store seasonal clothing, line the bottom of the suitcase with acid-free tissue and use sheets to wrap each garment for additional protection. The bottom of the closet can be used for storing large pieces of sports equipment such as golf clubs or seasonal pieces such as winter boots and galoshes. When storing these items, make sure that they're clean and dry and not touching the coats within the closet. And if at all possible, keep some space with a few empty hangers to hang your guests' coats when they come to visit. Who wants to have their coat thrown on their friend's bed or chair only to discover that Fluffy or Mittens has been using it as a personal bed for the last few hours?

If you have a large collection of winter coats, why not consider using off-site storage when you're not using them? Many dry cleaners offer clothing storage as part of their service to customers. And don't forget the joys of donating or consigning clothing that we discussed in chapter 3.

THE KIDS' CLOSET

Like your closet, your children's closets should be used for storing and displaying clothing. And because children's clothes are much smaller than adult-sized items, triple rods can be used to maximize the space within your children's closets.

Organize clothes in a child's closet in the same way you organize your own wardrobe. Hang like with like, and separate garments by color. If your child has a favorite outfit that he or she wears as an ensemble, hang those pieces together to encourage your child to dress him- or herself. An organized closet will also make it easier for your children to find what they want to wear and let them make wardrobe choices with as little fuss as possible. And most important, it will avoid the "Where is my shirt? Where are my pants?" routine that plagues many homes every morning.

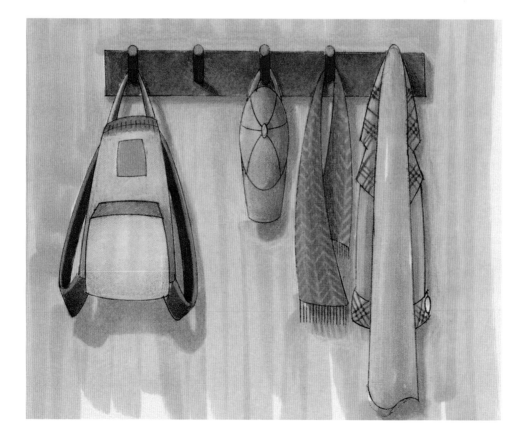

The standard child's hanger is 12 inches wide. Make sure to buy hangers of all the same material and encourage your children to properly hang up their clothing. The mantra "No wire hangers" comes into play and helps your children take pride in caring for their clothes so that they always look their best.

Play Hook-y

A set of hooks or a peg rail is a great way to encourage your child to keep his or her closet tidy by hanging things such as pajamas, sweatshirts, and hoodies that don't require a hanger. Also, this is the perfect spot for your kid to hang a backpack or book bag so that you can avoid the daily hunt for this elusive item as the school bus sits in front of the house honking its horn. Shoes, boots, and other footwear can be stored on a small shoe shelf in the bottom of the closet. Encourage your child to keep footwear in pairs and in good repair.

Storing Toys, Sporting Equipment, and Dance/ Exercise Clothes

Every kid has lots of stuff that needs to be stowed. Toys should be kept in toy boxes or storage bins in the child's room. However, toy overflow can be kept in storage boxes or in cubbies in the bottom of the child's closet. Like clothing, toys should be edited and cleaned out every six months to a year, as many children's playthings are designed for age-appropriateness. If your child has outgrown some toys, give them away or donate them to your favorite charity. Many towns have consignment shops exclusively dedicated to children, so check the phone directory or the Internet if you'd like

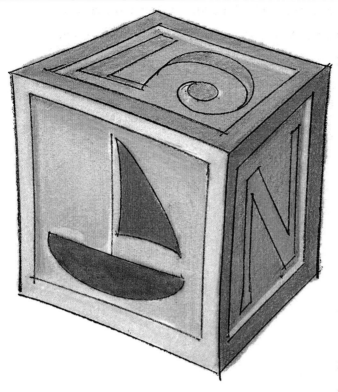

to consign some of your children's items. Throw away any toys that are broken, damaged, incomplete, or soiled. Trust me, you'll never find the missing piece to the jigsaw puzzle of a snowstorm in the Arctic. Throw it away!

Like toys, sporting equipment can be kept in bins in the child's closet. Never put away any sporting equipment that is wet or dirty as it can encourage mold, mildew, or insect infestation. Also, encourage your child to put dirty uniforms and jerseys in a clothing hamper or laundry bag. The laundry bag or clothing hamper should be located in a spot where it can be easily accessed and emptied on a frequent basis. Try not to keep the laundry bag or hamper in the closet, because its contents can stink up the clothes being stored there. Dancing and sports items such as leotards, tights, shorts, ballet slippers, and so on can be kept on a shelf or in a bin that's easy for your child to reach. If your child uses a gym, sports, or dance bag, encourage the child to empty it after every rehearsal, practice, or game. Never use these types of bags, to store dirty stuff.

We've cleaned, organized, hung up and folded all the items in the various closets throughout your home. Now we're ready for the last section of the book: "Staying Organized." Turn to the next chapter to begin your day-to-day maintenance program of your closets.

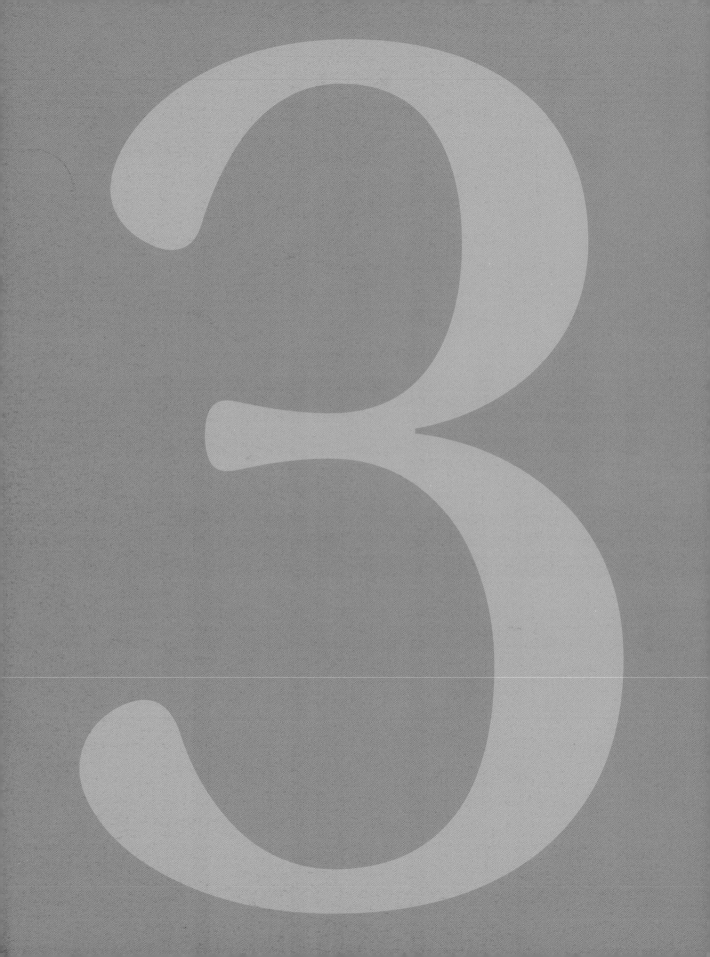

STAYING
ORGANIZED

You've done it! Your closets are organized, everything is perfectly folded and appropriately hung (on the right hanger in the right order), and you are able to actually shop your closet. After all your hard work, now's the time to talk about how to maintain your closets and wardrobe. Keep it neat. Keep it clean. Keep it organized. The hard part is over; you have achieved closet nirvana. Read on to see what to do to maintain this tranquil wardrobe refuge.

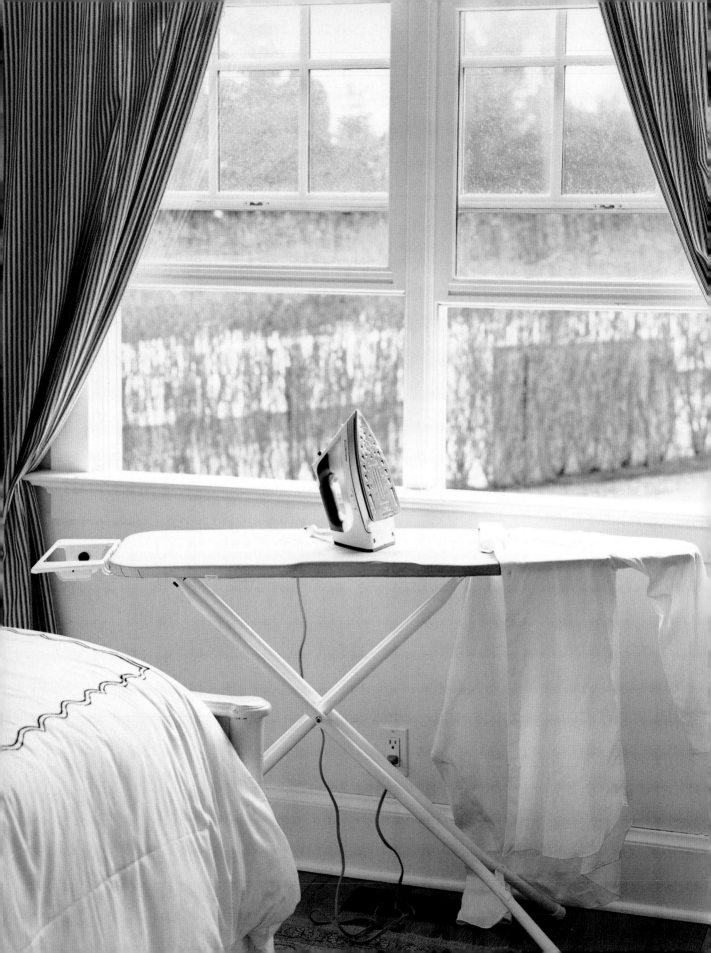

CHAPTER 8

Day-to-Day Maintenance

LITTLE THINGS MEAN A LOT

To keep your closet looking its best, you have to establish a routine that becomes part of your daily drill. I travel a great deal to my New York office, my Florida office, and to various clients around the country. I have established a routine that lets me get ready in a flash and keeps my home looking tidy and peaceful. Do what I do: When you get ready for bed at night, don't leave your clothes in a pile on the floor or flung all over your room. Designate a specific chair or location—such as a clothes rack, dresser top, or bench—where you can put things that need to be stored in the closet. Then when you get up in the morning, you can hang the previous day's outfit up before picking your clothes for that day. Do this every night and day. Or if you're now becoming a total neat freak, you can actually put away your clothes before you retire for the evening. Whatever method works for you, properly store whatever you have previously worn before you pull out a new outfit from your closet. Do not allow clothes to pile up on the chair or dresser top. Not only does this unsightly mess create a frat-house ambience but it also exposes your clothes to potential dangers. Unsightly and hard-to-remove wrinkles can appear, ensemble pieces can be mislaid or lost, your dog or cat can nest in your favorite outfits and leave dander and hair all over them, and mystery stains or tears can occur. Don't let this happen. Put your things away. The result is a tidy room and an organized closet that is a source of comfort and serenity in this chaotic world.

THE IRON AGE

With the availability of wrinkle-free clothes and the abundance of synthetic fibers, many people think that ironing is a lost art. It is not! There is nothing more unappealing than seeing a person walking down the street in a wrinkled suit, showing up for a job interview in a wrinkled dress, or going on a date with a wrinkled shirt! Not only does that person look sloppy but also the image that it presents says, *I don't care about my appearance.* This makes the viewer think, *Hmmm. If this person doesn't care about their appearance, what else are they not paying attention to?* So hang up your clothes properly on the appropriate style of hanger to keep them shipshape. For quick touch-ups, invest in a decent clothing steamer. These can be purchased for anywhere from as little as $29 for a handheld travel model to more than $100 for a large professional one; they're available at many different types of retailers. However, there is nothing like a

SHOP YOUR CLOSET

good old-fashioned iron and ironing board to keep your clothes pressed and sharp-looking. Personally, I hate ironing, so I steam everything. My secret is to use two-thirds distilled water to one-third lavender linen water in my steamer. This results in wrinkle-free clothes, and I save a lot of money on dry-cleaning bills. However, if you absolutely hate to iron or refuse to steam, your dry cleaner or local laundromat or laundry center offers pressing and ironing services for a fee.

ironing 101—how to iron a shirt

1. Read the label to find out what type of material the shirt is made of. If it's cotton, set your iron on high; if it's a polyester–cotton blend, use a medium setting. If the shirt is made of silk, acetate, polyester, nylon, rayon, or any type of acrylic, use the low setting to avoid scorching or melting. Linen water (scented or unscented) or regular tap water that's sprinkled on the shirt or placed in your iron, if it's a steam model, will make wrinkles disappear more easily. Spray starch, available at any supermarket, can be used if a supercrisp starched look is what you want. Some people don't like to sprinkle water on their clothes as they're ironing, for fear of scorching. A good alternative is to place your

shirt in your freezer for a few hours prior to ironing it. The shirt absorbs moisture from the freezer, resulting in a smoother ironing experience.

2. Place the shirt facedown on the ironing board or on a flat surface (such as a tabletop, bed, or countertop). If it's the latter, put a towel or piece of thick cotton fabric on top to protect the tabletop from scorching and prevent the shirt from sticking to the surface of your make-do ironing board. Iron the back of the collar first, then the front. Iron from the edges in, in smooth strokes.

3. Iron the cuffs of each sleeve (make sure they are unbuttoned), first the inside and then the outside. Iron each sleeve.

4. Flip the shirt over, place one of the front panels flat on the board, and iron the entire panel.

5. Pull the shirt over the board, positioning the back of the shirt flat on the surface. Iron the back of the shirt. Once this is finished, iron the remaining front panel.

6. Immediately hang the warm shirt on an appropriate hanger to avoid wrinkling.

7. Irons get very hot. Never leave a hot iron unattended. Never leave an iron facedown while it is plugged in and unattended for any length of time. Be careful when using an iron around children or pets.

SHOP YOUR CLOSET

THE CLEAN MACHINE

Repeat after me; "I will throw dirty clothes in the hamper, laundry bag, or dry-cleaning bag." There, wasn't that easy? Who wants to look at dirty clothes scattered all around your house? The easiest solution is to purchase a closed hamper (one that comes complete with a lid) that discretely fits into your home's décor. Available in every imaginable style and type of material, this basic can be found at your favorite home-furnishings store, department store, or even your supermarket or drugstore. The closed hamper is the most convenient and simplest way to eliminate dirty laundry from your sight. Divide the hamper so one side can be used to store your dry cleaning and the other for laundry. Never place dirty clothes in a pile on your floor or, God forbid, rehang them in your closet. If you do, then when it comes time to look for an outfit to put on, you won't have a clue if what you want to wear is clean or dirty. And even worse, dirty clothing can invite unwanted insects into your closet, not to mention an amazing assortment of smells. Do not allow your closet to become an insect smorgasbord. Moth larva will happily chew holes in your favorite cashmere sweater, roaches will seek the smallest drops of moisture and bits of food for nourishment, and . . . I'm getting grossed

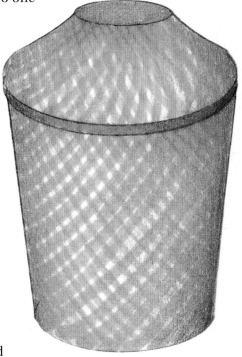

out just thinking about it; I think you get the picture. If you leave soiled items unattended in your closet, not only does the potential for insect infestation exist but also you face the threat of permanent staining of your beloved clothing.

We all sweat and sometimes we have the occasional spill or grooming mishap or inadvertently drop bits of our lunch or dinner on our shirts or jackets. If this happens, bring these items to your dry cleaner as soon as possible and specify what stained your favorite silk blouse or fantastic wool skirt.

A good dry cleaner is familiar with the three basic types of stains: earth-based stains (fruit juices, chocolate, wine, coffee, and tea, for example), protein-based stains (this group includes dairy products and blood), and oil-based stains (including vegetable oils, mayonnaise, make-up, lipstick, and motor oil). Don't try to treat or wash the spot yourself, as rubbing or applying untested cleaners, water, or anything else to the area can result in permanently setting the stain. Leave it to the pros!

cleaning and care of clothing

Dry Cleaning When cleaning clothing, always check the garment's label for cleaning instructions as supplied by the manufacturer. If the label says "dry-clean only" or "dry-cleaning recommended," take the garment to your favorite dry cleaners.

Laundering If clothing can be laundered, read the instructions for wash-water temperature and for preferred drying method—line drying, flat drying, or machine drying. Wash darks, whites, and light-colored clothes separately. For colorfastness and

TO EVERYTHING THERE IS A SEASON

Surprise! The seasons affect your closet. Those days of hanging your favorite ski parka next to your favorite one-piece bathing suit are over. When you change your closet over to the appropriate season, it allows you to do two things: First, it gives you the opportunity to make sure that whatever season's clothes you're done with for the year are properly cleaned, maintained, and carefully stored so that when you need them next year, they are ready to wear. Second, the seasons provide you with the invaluable opportunity of doing a mini inventory of what you need to replenish or change in your wardrobe. If, as they do for me, the words *end-of-season sale* bring a smile to your lips and put a song in your heart, this is when you can shop for those items you've been missing. You can buy what you need to fill those fashion holes and then put your new purchases away for the following year's season. How cool is that? Not only will you be secure in the knowledge that your wardrobe is complete and ready when you need it but also you will have saved yourself a lot of money by shopping during peak sale season.

recommended cleaning products—that is, bleach—check the label. If you are unsure of a piece of clothing's colorfastness, wash it separately in cold water, using a mild detergent. Avoid using bleach on dark clothes, as it can remove dyes and result in permanent color damage. When doing a wash, fill the machine with water, add your detergent, and then add the wash load. Never pour detergent directly onto clothing, as it may stain.

seasons change and so should your closet

* When changing over your closet from one season to the next, give yourself enough time to properly complete the task. Set aside an evening after work or a Saturday or Sunday to get this done. You'll be glad you did.

* Examine each garment and repair or mend as needed. If a shirt is missing a button, sew it on. If your boots are scuffed, polish them. If your zipper is broken on your ski jacket, fix it or have the shoe-repair shop replace it.

* Before your pack it away, clean it! Bring whatever needs to be dry-cleaned to the dry cleaners and throw in the washing machine whatever needs to be laundered. Wash your swimsuits and beach wraps. Launder your shorts and tank tops. Dry-clean your favorite wool coat and cashmere scarf. Don't put anything away that has not been cleaned. Remember, your closet is not an insect smorgasbord, nor do you want to pull out your favorite ski sweater only to discover a big stain across the front.

* If you are lucky enough to have a seasonal closet, use it to store heavy winter clothing and coats. Attics and basements can also be used, but make certain that these spaces do not get hot or wet. Heat and moisture are natural enemies of your clothing. To avoid water damage, use a rubber mat or tarp from your favorite home-improvement store, such as Lowe's or Home Depot, to cover the floor. Also, large plastic bins or boxes (like the ones from Rubbermaid and available at many stores and retailers) are perfect for storing these items in these locations.

SHOP YOUR CLOSET

We've cleaned, organized, maintained, and seasonalized your closets. Now you're ready to make your closet work for you! Say good-bye to frustrating hours of trying to find what clothes to pack for your vacation, only to discover after you've arrived at your destination that you forgot half of what you needed to bring! Turn to the next chapter, *"From Closet to Suitcase,"* to see how your well-organized closet makes travel preparations easier and reduces the stress of getting ready for a trip.

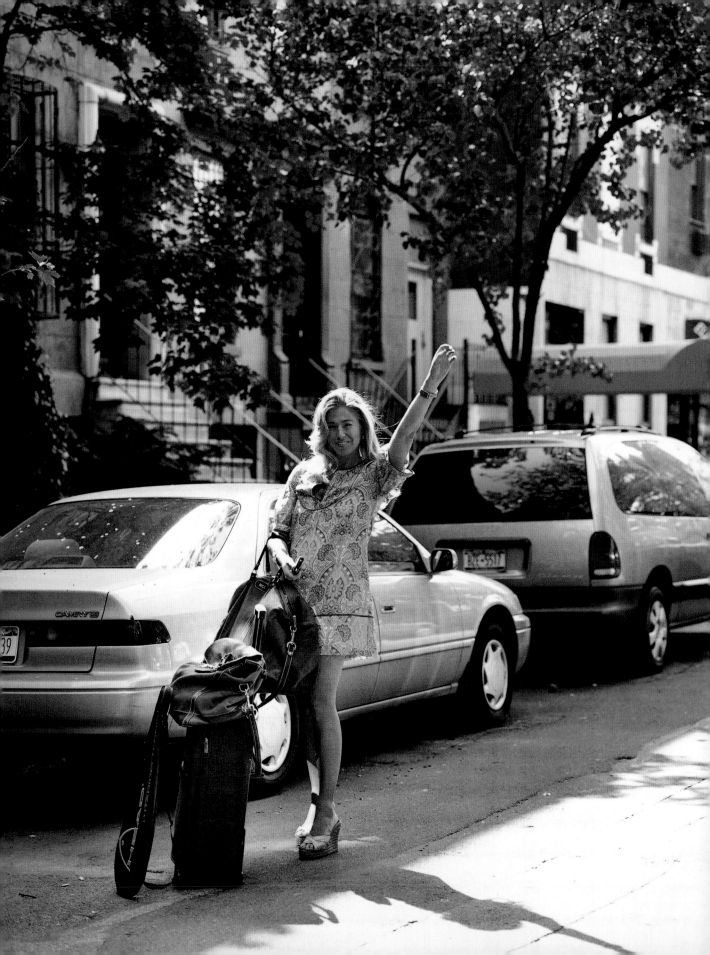

CHAPTER 9

From Closet to Suitcase

Packing. The word is enough to make the strongest of us weak in the knees. Do you ask yourself these questions every time you prepare to leave for a trip: Where are the suitcases? How much should I bring? How do I pack so that my clothes don't arrive looking as if they were slept in for a month? What should I carry on in case my suitcase gets lost or misplaced?

Fear not. Your organized, easy-to-shop closet will make packing a headache-free snap. No longer will you have to dig through piles of clothes to find your bathing suit, wrestle your suitcase from the abyss of your closet, or face clumps of disorganized clothing on mismatched hangers. Your wardrobe is at the ready for any type of trip. If you follow the useful tips given here, packing for your next trip will be a nonevent. So take advantage of those reduced airfares and allow yourself to be whisked away on a last-minute vacation. Your closets are organized and you are ready!

YOU BIG LUG—BUYING THE RIGHT LUGGAGE

Buying the right luggage can make the difference between the trip from hell and a lighthearted skip through the airport, train station, or bus terminal. Before buying any suitcase, Pullman, garment bag, backpack, tote, duffle bag, or carry-on, consider the following:

* *How much do I want to spend?* Like anything else, buy the best that you can afford. A $9.95 suitcase may seem like the bargain of the century, but the old adage "You get what you pay for" comes into play. Cheap is cheap, and crap is crap. Buy the best that you can. Not only will it perform better but it also will last longer.

* *How am I going to use it?* If you want a suitcase that can be used for any type of trip, from a quick weekend getaway to a three-week cruise, buy one that has the capability to meet your needs. Does it have a lot of compartments to store various things? Does it have wheels to make for easy transportation? Does it have a sturdy retractable handle for easy pulling? Does it come with a shoulder strap so I can carry it on my shoulder if the need arises? Does it fit into a standard overhead compartment on an airplane, bus, or train so I can carry it onboard and avoid the possibility of its getting lost? Consider these factors to find the right model.

* *What is it made of, and how much does it weigh?* Those old-fashioned oversized, hard-sided suitcases were rugged; they could be dropped from amazing heights and jumped on by 800-pound gorillas. (Remember those old commercials, or am I dating myself?) But they weighed a ton. These days, many prefer the ease of carrying on. A 50-pound suitcase you have to schlep through security checkpoints and that doesn't fit into an

overhead compartment or under your seat adds to your stress level and creates a host of health issues, from a strained back to aching arm muscles. Buy the lightest model possible that makes for easy transportation but is sturdy enough to withstand the rigors of travel. If you are checking your luggage, think about the bag handlers who load and unload an airplane. Let's just say that the words *gentle* and *careful* do not come into play. Have you ever seen a suitcase burst open, spilling its entire contents on the baggage carousel, leaving the poor traveler scrambling to gather up underwear, socks, clothing, and toiletries? Get a light, sturdy bag and one that's made from a durable, easily cleaned material that doesn't show too much scuffing or dirt.

suitcase

101

Today, there is a huge assortment of luggage available at your favorite store, online, or in a catalogue. Luggage can be broken down into the following categories: large suitcases and Pullmans, trunks, carry-ons, business cases/computer cases, duffle bags, totes, garment bags and carriers, and backpacks.

Large Suitcases and Pullmans There are three types of luggage in the category of large suitcases and Pullmans—hard-sided, semisoft, and soft-sided. These can range in size from 24 to 36 inches. Hard-sided suitcases usually feature wheels, handles, locks, and pull straps and are extremely durable in the face of wear and tear. They can be constructed of various materials, including plastic, metal, and synthetic molded materials. Some feature interior frame construction of wood or metal and have a soft covering of leather, nylon, and fabric (either synthetic, such as polyester, or natural, such as cotton or silk). Semisoft suitcases allow for some expansion room in packing and usually have wheels and pull straps or shoulder straps to assist in transport. Soft-sided suitcases are made of a synthetic or natural fabric (they can be nylon, polyester, leather, canvas, cotton, and so on) to allow for easy expansion and to handle various size loads. They have zipper closures and stiffeners instead of an interior framework. Special note: you can buy suitcases in matching sets of different sizes to ready you for whatever type or trip you may need to take.

Trunks Think old-time steamship/luxury cruise liner travel (the *Queen Elizabeth 2*) or summer camp. Trunks are large rectangular or square boxes that come in varying sizes and materials and are excellent for transporting huge amounts of clothing or delicate instruments and breakables such as Grandma's china, photography equipment, or priceless art. These sturdy forms of luggage are also extremely heavy and usually require two people to carry them.

Carry-Ons Versatile time-savers, carry-ons are small enough to stow under an airplane seat or in the overhead compartment (the bag usually has to be 22 inches wide or less for this). They can be made of varying materials and hard, like suitcases (think Doris Day traveling on the train with her makeup case), semisoft, or soft. Always use a carry-on to transport important documents (passports, identification, tickets) and things such as prescription medications,

SHOP YOUR CLOSET

eyeglasses, jewelry, and extra cash and/or credit cards.

Business/Computer Cases Business or computer cases can hold your business papers and necessities and your laptop computer or other electronic devices. Built-in padding in computer cases helps prevent shock, so you can avoid damage to your expensive electronic gadgets. Briefcases come in a variety of materials and, like carry-ons, can be hard, semisoft, or soft. For overnight business trips, they are an excellent way to schlep your work, as well as a quick change of casual clothing.

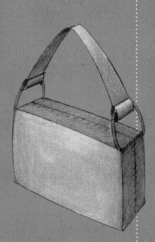

Duffle Bags Big and roomy duffles (think Popeye the Sailor) are a great way to carry a large amount of clothing. They're usually made of fabric (natural or synthetic) and have large shoulder straps, or sometimes wheels, for easy transport.

Totes The simple tote bag comes in a variety of sizes, shapes, and materials and is a convenient way to carry your necessities. Some styles have pockets to segregate smaller items and oversized straps to allow the bag to slip onto your shoulder for easier carrying.

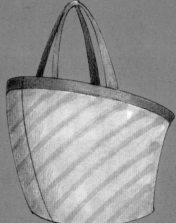

Garment Bags Garment bags are wonderful travel buddies for carrying suits, dresses, and any garments that you store by hanging. They usually can be brought onboard a plane and hung in the plane's closet to avoid wrinkling their contents. Typically designed to hold two to four items, they can be made of many different types of material and range in length from 40 to 60 inches.

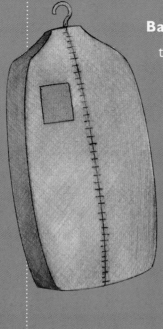

Backpacks Designed for more casual traveling or outdoor trips (think college students in Europe or campers hiking the Appalachian Trail), backpacks are a good way to carry what you need while keeping your arms and hands free. Because these are carried on your back, be sure to try on any you're considering buying to test their fit and feel. Backpacks come with either metal frames or no frames (depending on how much weight and what you need to carry) and are usually made of nylon, canvas, or leather.

Whatever type or style of luggage you purchase, check its construction to ensure that it will be able to withstand numerous trips. I remember one harrowing business trip; I was running to get a connecting flight at Chicago's O'Hare International Airport when my Pullman literally exploded clothing and stuff all over the floor. My life was literally laid out for all of my fellow travelers to see. I had to quickly scoop everything up into my arms, run into the nearest gift shop, and buy the most ghastly plastic tote emblazoned with the immortal words "Chicago, the Windy City." So when I landed in Los Angeles, I walked off the plane looking ravishing and carrying my trip's worth of clothing jammed into my $5.95 (on sale) piece of fabulous luggage. This experience taught me to really look at the quality of a piece of luggage before buying it. You don't want to get caught the way I did.

Look for reinforced seams, tightly woven fabrics for strength, frames that are wrapped to avoid damaging clothing, interior straps to hold piles of clothing firmly in place, recessed handles (which are less likely to be damaged than nonrecessed ones), wide-track wheels recessed into the frame of the bag to prevent its tipping while you're pulling it, and large zippers with big pulls to make for easier closing and opening. Finally, choose a color that will not show dirt or scuffing easily—and mark your luggage with a distinctive piece of tape, ribbon, or marking for easy identification.

PACK IT IN

You have the right piece of luggage and you're ready to pack your stuff and dash off to the airport for your well-deserved weekend away. But now you're wondering what to bring and how to pack it so it doesn't look as if you wore your entire suitcase contents on the plane. Read on to learn the fine art of packing.

The rule of thumb when packing for a trip is "pack everything you think you're going to need and then reduce it by half." How often have you gone on a trip and packed enough outfits to clothe half the resort? How many sweaters did you pack for that ski trip, only to realize that you wore the same two for the entire week, while the rest were snugly ensconced in your room at the lodge? If you're going away for a weekend, bring separates that can be mixed and matched to create various outfits with completely different looks. A crewneck sweater worn over a blouse and jeans is a great casual look for a day of shopping or sightseeing. That same outfit can be glamorized for a night out on the town by simply replacing the jeans with a flouncy skirt and taking off the sweater and adding a silk scarf or fabulous necklace and earrings for a little touch of evening glimmer. Longer trips call for more outfits, but you don't have to pack your entire closet. Many things can be worn more than once (unless, of course, you're trekking through the rain forests of the Amazon), and often, destination spots offer dry-cleaning and laundry services at a nominal charge. Or do your own laundry at a local wash center, or drop off your dry cleaning at a local establishment. If all else fails and you're desperate for something different or (gasp!) clean, go shopping!

what to pack for a weekend getaway

If you're going away for the weekend, here's what to pack:

* *Men:* Something to sleep in (if desired), two changes of underwear, two pairs of socks, a pair of jeans, a T-shirt or casual shirt, a sport/dress shirt, a sweater, dress slacks (if needed), a tie (if needed), a sports jacket, a pair of shoes, and toiletries/grooming aids.
* *Women:* Something to sleep in (if desired), two changes of underwear, two pairs of socks, jeans, a T-shirt or casual shirt, a dressy shirt or blouse, dress slacks or skirt (if needed), dressy shoes or pumps, panty hose, jewelry (if desired), silk scarf (if desired), and toiletries/grooming aids.

We've got everything ready to pack; now how do we pack it so that it stays fresh, clean, and as wrinkle-free as possible? First, pack heavier things such as jeans, sweaters, sweatshirts, and jackets neatly folded in the bottom of the suitcase. Then pack shirts, dresses, dress slacks/pants, and skirts on top. More easily wrinkled items should be placed at the bottom of the pile, with less-wrinkle-prone stuff toward the top. With shirts, fold the sleeves in toward the torso and fold the bottom half up to create a nice rectangle. Stack shirts neatly and snugly on top of one another in nice bundles. Lay dresses over the open suitcase, so that the ends hang over the sides, and gently fold them into the suitcase. Pants and skirts should be folded in half lengthwise and then folded in half to reduce the amount of wrinkling.

To pack accessories, roll ties and belts and place in pockets to avoid shifting. Acid-free tissue is great for wrapping around ties to prevent soil-

SHOP YOUR CLOSET

ing or damage. Pack underwear in mesh laundry bags or side pockets to save space. When packing shoes, put them in plastic or cloth shoe bags. (Some shoes come with them; if not, purchase them at organizational stores or housewares stores). Place them along the perimeter of your suitcase to take up as little space as possible, individually bagged and placed heel to toe. Also, use your socks to stuff your shoes. This will save room in your suitcase and help your shoes retain their shape while traveling. Fine lingerie, silk scarves, and panty hose should be placed in lingerie bags to prevent snagging and bunching. Toiletries should be securely capped and wrapped in individual plastic bags that can be sealed to prevent leakage and then placed in a separate toiletries bag. Nobody wants to arrive at their destination only to discover that their bottle of shampoo has opened and drowned their favorite clothes in a pool of sticky green liquid! Essential toiletries (toothbrush, toothpaste, deodorant, makeup, and medication) should be packed into your carry-on in case your suitcase is lost or stolen. Also, *never* pack jewelry, cash, identification, passports, keys, travel documents, credit cards, or anything else valuable in your suitcase. Always pack these items in your carry-on for safekeeping. The most wonderful vacation will turn into the trip from hell if you lose your suitcase packed with all of your travel documents, identification, and money. Don't let this happen to you. Pack smart and travel safe!

Picture this: Your closets are amazing! You're all set to travel at a moment's notice; you've addressed all your closet and wardrobe needs. But just when you thought it was all smooth sailing from here, a significant other arrives on the scene. Where do you put his or her stuff? How do you make room for their wardrobe? What are you going to do? Breathe. It's okay. Turn to the next chapter and discover "What to Do When He (or She) Moves In."

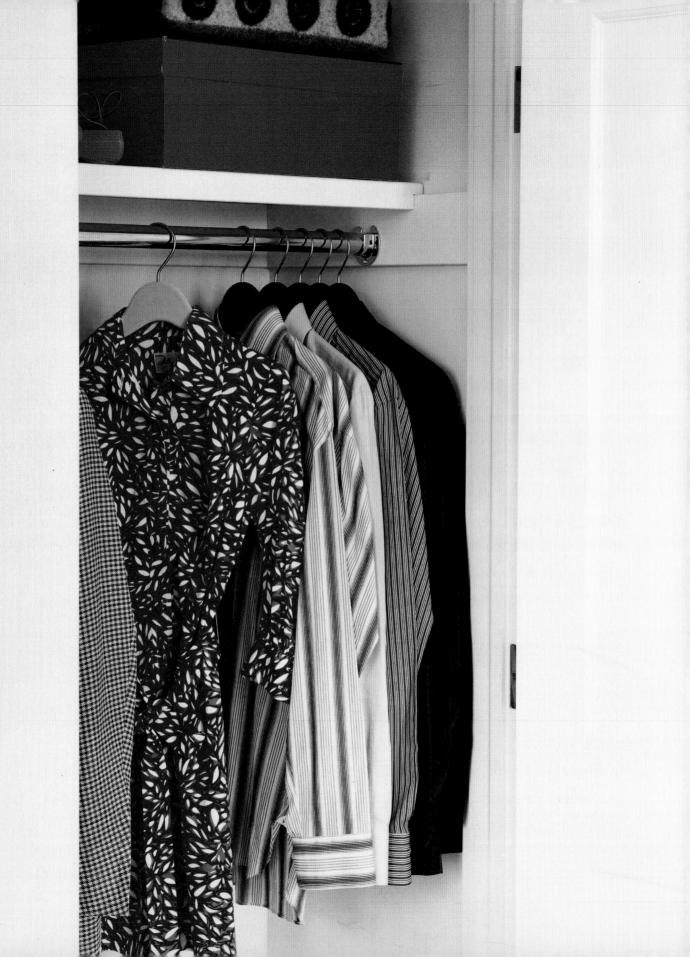

CHAPTER 10

What to Do When He (or She) Moves In

Life is good. Your closets are organized, your seasonal stuff is put away, your shelves neatly display your shoes, your handbags are hanging on hooks, and your sweaters are neatly folded and easy to view. Then, the unexpected happens. You meet Mr. or Ms. Right and you start to date. The dating becomes serious and you start to date exclusively. Next, you both begin talking "commitment speak." Now, it's Friday night and tomorrow (yes, *tomorrow*) your committed significant other (SO) is moving in and (gasp!) bringing along all their stuff. What now? You've learned how to be your own editor, discovering the joys and benefits of taking stock, and it shows. However, certain unavoidable problems pop up when your beloved arrives on the scene with all of their stuff. Let's begin to handle this situation and discuss how to deal with his humongous tie collection and her endless array of dresses.

My husband Jon and I met at our mutual friend's wedding in Switzerland. We became fast friends and started dating. Four and a half months into our courtship, we decided to get married and eloped at city hall. Before I realized it, I had a new husband and roommate in my one-bedroom loft with its one little closet that was barely big enough for me and my stuff, let alone a six-foot one-inch man who had enough clothes to make us finding a storage solution seem like *Mission Impossible.* Yes, we are planning on buying a bigger apartment, but that is not in our plans for another year or two, and my one-bedroom apartment is way too good a deal to let slip away, so we knew we had to make it work. So I went to work. I gathered together my crackerjack team from Clos-ette, and we transformed a not-enough closet for one into a closet built for two. Now, I know you're thinking, *What's the big deal? She owns a closet design/organizational business, so it was a piece of cake.* Well, it wasn't. I don't own my apartment (it's a great rental), and I found out it's not so easy to practice what you preach. But I managed it, and the result is fantastic! We came up with some simple solutions that were cost-effective and practical. First, I edited my wardrobe and my husband's. I thought *I* was a pack rat! We got rid of the older clothes that he was hanging on to for God knows why, and we streamlined his quantitatively huge (he had a lot!) shirt and tie collection. Second, we use the same style hangers for our clothing. It keeps the look uniform and neat and makes it easier to hang things up and put things away. Third, we built a double-hanging, three-sided closet/armoire out of inexpensive plywood (that we painted) and used maple boards to trim it out. This three-sided armoire sits proudly in the corner of the master bedroom and looks really good. Fourth, we added another chest of drawers to give him drawer and seasonal storage (you have to put those ski sweaters somewhere). Finally, I took the pledge to stop shopping so much and even edit my thoughts of bingeing. I needed to embrace my new limited space, and my new husband-partner-roommate needed to be able to feel that he

SHOP YOUR CLOSET

had ownership in the apartment and a say about how his wardrobe should be stored and maintained.

COEDIT TO COEXIST

You did it for yourself. Now it's time to assist your SO with the editing of their wardrobe. If you're afraid that this discussion might turn into a full-fledged World War III, complete with personal ambushes such as "How can one person have two hundred sweaters?" then enlist the aid of a mutual friend. A third party can help smooth the transition of incorporating a new wardrobe into the space that yours currently occupies. You don't want to make this individual the "monkey in the middle," but their input may help avoid arguments between the two of you and provide another perspective that is not entwined with your agenda or your SO's agenda. Also, don't forget to share with your new cohabitant the joys of donating (a great tax write-off), consigning (extra money in their pocket), and giving away (fuzzy, warm feeling for all humankind) clothes that they no longer wear, want, or like.

Don't allow their boxes to grow like an invading alien army taking over your home. You have come too far and have accomplished too much to go back to your old haphazard ways. So if they start storing their shoes in the oven, hanging their coats behind the curtains, and putting their sweaters in the bathroom because they have no where else to put them, don't be alarmed. Stay calm. Consider what to do to stem the tide of clothing chaos and put your plan into action. Be brave. Be strong. And most important, be fair, realizing that you may have to do a finer edit of your own wardrobe.

Designer Lara Meiland of Lara Hélène Bridal Atelier on Madison Avenue in New York City remembers when her husband, Claude Shaw, moved in:

We did a lot of editing when we moved in together, but that being said, when I said, "I do," I had visions of partnership and sharing in mind, but unfortunately for my new husband, when it came to divvying up closet space in our new loft apartment, I became ruthless. I allocated a closet in a separate bedroom for Claude and took control of both the walk-in and the reach-in closets in the master bedroom. I justified this in my mind by convincing myself that he needed his own personal space and he approved of my shopping habit. This was a very tricky task, but I managed it and remain guilt free to this day. Then again, I do own a bridal store, Lara Hélène, on the Upper East Side of Manhattan. (Let's face it—being located on Madison Avenue is a tough place to be for a shopaholic like me.) I personally think that the level of delicacy with which this situation must be dealt is proportional to how long a couple has been together. My husband and I have been together for five years, so I think he knew what to expect. For my impassioned friends who recently eloped (Melanie, that's you and Jon), the negotiations may take a bit more time and may require concessions from both sides.

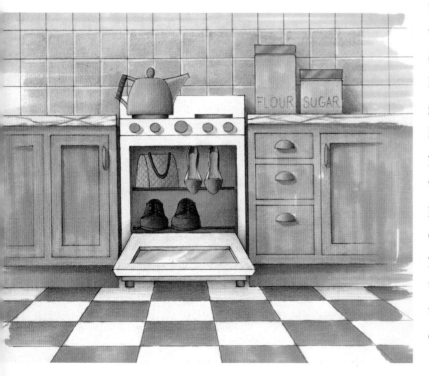

SHOP YOUR CLOSET

HAVE NO FEAR, STORAGE IS HERE

Storage can be your best friend. As we discussed earlier, store your off-season clothes off-site at your favorite dry cleaners. Store your SO's there as well. If you find that there's a lot more stuff than your dry cleaner can handle, or if other stuff, such as their favorite childhood bicycle, 50 boxes of college textbooks, and an endless collection of beer cans, threatens your home's serenity and your sanity, consider the beauty of self-storage. To find a secure storage facility in your neighborhood, check with friends and neighbors for recommendations. Do your homework and research the ones listed with your local chamber of commerce or that are members of the Better Business Bureau. The Internet and your local phone directory are also great sources for finding storage possibilities.

Before hauling any precious belongings to an unknown location, do the legwork. Pay a visit to the facilities you're considering. Meet with the management and ask to review their contract to see what terms apply to people leasing space from them. Also, find out how often rates increase, what can or cannot be stored in the location, the hours and days of access, who has access, what security measures are in place, how easy it is to add or remove stuff from the storage unit, how far it is from your home, and how easy it is to get to. Look around and see where this business is located and what the neighborhood is like. Is there a secure place to park your car while loading and unloading, or if you don't drive, is the facility located near a convenient form of mass transit (bus, train, subway) or a taxi stand? Don't forget to ask if the company offers help in lugging stuff in and out, if it have means of disposing of garbage, if it has elevators to move things to higher floors or whether you have to climb stairs, and what type of insurance it carries in case of a disaster that damages your stuff (including fire, theft, flood, and acts of nature or humankind). Find out if any penalties exist if you break your lease and what happens if you and your SO break up and how this will affect the contract. Don't forget to ask what happens to your stuff if you miss a payment, and any other scenarios that come to mind. Being thorough and asking some very pointed questions will provide you with peace of mind and reduce the possibility of head-aches and stress later on.

TIMES THEY ARE A-CHANGIN'—AND SO IS YOUR CLOSET

When you designed your closet for your wardrobe, you looked at the space as if it was a single unit. Now, take everything out and view it with a new set of eyes. Instead of seeing it as a closet built for one, you are now the proud owner of a closet built for two. Such simple solutions as changing closet rods or adding some additional shelf space can make a world of dif-ference.

Just as you did when you were setting up and organizing your closet for your wardrobe, look to see what needs your SO has in terms of their wardrobe—do they have suits that need to be hung, sweaters that need to be folded, and shoes that require shelf space? Review their clothing in combination with yours and design accordingly.

Peg rails (long pieces of wood with wooden pegs sticking out of them), tie racks, storage bins, and extra shelves can provide the perfect place for him or her to hang their belts, display their ties, store their scarves, and hook their handbags. Be creative, and remember, as much as you need to shop your closet to get dressed and ready for the day ahead, so do they!

SEPARATE BUT EQUAL

Even if you and your honey are sharing a closet, you should each have your own area designated to store your clothes. Do not try to commingle your wardrobes. It won't work. Your dresses hanging next to his shirts, intermixed with your skirts and his pants, will only create confusion, chaos, and frustration. You can hang your things in the same closet, but keep things separate.

If you have more than one closet in your home, designate one as yours and one as theirs. This simple solution allows each of you to have your own private wardrobe space and keep it as you like it. Let's face it: some of us are born neat freaks and some of us are born slobs. Separate closets can be the saving grace in your relationship if you have differing approaches to your wardrobe. If you do not have two closets, perhaps you can bring in a freestanding wardrobe or armoire. As we learned in chapter 4, any freestanding wardrobe can be fitted with shelves, rods, or a combination of the two to accommodate various clothing pieces. If you're not a tool lover like Bob Vila and you think Home Depot is the train station in the town where you come from, then use a handy man or carpenter to custom fit your wardrobe for whatever clothes it will hold. And if you ever break up, then after he or she leaves, you can turn the wardrobe into an off-season clothing closet for yourself or convert it into something fabulous like a private bar or a television cabinet!

Our next chapter, "Beyond the Closet," shows how everything you've learned from this book can be easily adapted where storage problems and needs exist. From your CD collection to your medicine cabinet, from your pantry to your bookshelves, read on to find out how to organize and streamline these troublesome areas within your home.

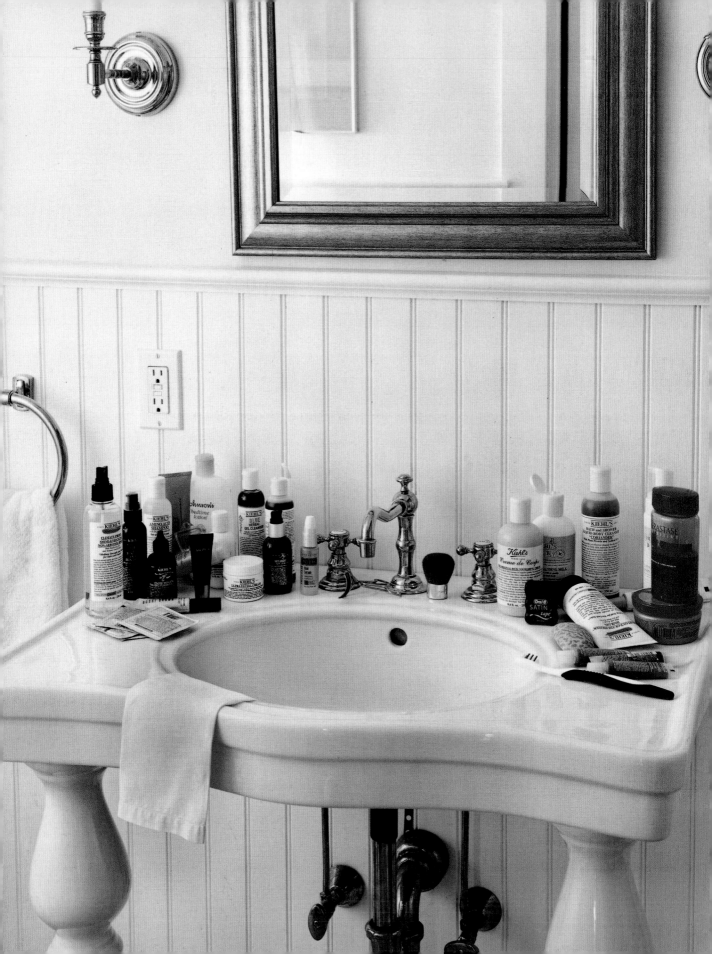

CHAPTER 11

Beyond the Closet

Look at all we've learned and how far we've come since we started! Now let's use the basic principles of editing and organization that were applied to our closets and see if there are other areas in the home where these fundamentals can bring order to chaos and serenity to sloppiness.

THE MEDICINE CHEST

One of the most neglected spots in the home is the medicine chest. That all-important mini storage closet in our bathrooms that holds everything and helps to maintain our health and well-being, from toothpaste to tweezers to essential medications. Be honest—when was the last time you organized your medicine chest? Let's get started.

The first thing to do is empty the chest of all its contents. Throw out anything that's no longer usable—old toothbrushes, worn bars of soap, out-of-date prescription drugs, empty cough syrup bottles, and the like. Thoroughly clean the inside of the cabinet before returning anything to its shelves. Put less frequently used things on the top shelves and your daily stuff, such as shaving cream, razors, dental floss, and deodorant, on the lower shelves for easy access. Group like items together. By putting medicines and prescriptions on one shelf and grooming products on another, you'll find it easier to take stock of what you have and note what you need to buy. Always place items on the shelves with the labels or the front of the bottle facing out. This way, when you wander into the bathroom at the crack of dawn and grab something out of the medicine chest, you'll know you're brushing your teeth with toothpaste and not body lotion, hemorrhoid cream, or Nair.

TIP OF THE TRADE: Check use-by dates on grooming products, toiletries, over-the-counter medicines, and prescription drugs. Like food, these products, by law, must list a date by which they must be bought or used. If you can't find a date on a prescription medication bottle or remember when you purchased that antacid, the old adage "When in doubt, throw it out" should come into play. Also, when tossing unfinished over-the-counter medication, prescription drugs, or anything that can be harmful to children or pets or the environment, make certain it is properly disposed of. Don't throw these items into a bathroom wastebasket where inquisitive fingers and little snouts can easily find them. Avoid flushing medications down the toilet, as it's illegal in most communities. Before getting rid of any type of medication, find out from your local sanitation department or health officials how to handle it.

SOMEONE'S IN THE KITCHEN

Organizing your kitchen cabinets and food pantry will allow you to store your kitchen utensils, dishes, small appliances, and cookware more easily, as well as help you see what food items you have on hand and what you need to buy. How often do you start preparing your famous signature pasta dish for a dinner party only to discover that you don't have any dried oregano, the can of tomato paste you desperately need to finish your sauce turns out to be a can of tomato soup, and the box of spaghetti you wanted to use is half empty and looking a little beyond its prime?

The Pantry

As with your medicine chest, organize your food pantry by putting like with like. Store canned goods separately from boxed items. Stack larger stuff in the back of the pantry, with shorter things toward the front. Place pack-ages with the front or the label showing so that you can easily see what you have on hand. Anything that's been used should be properly resealed or put in a container with an airtight seal and stored according to the manufacturer's recommendations printed on the original packaging. If you transfer the contents to a glass or plastic container, be sure to put the name of the product on the outside, along with the use-by or sell-by date provided when you bought the item.

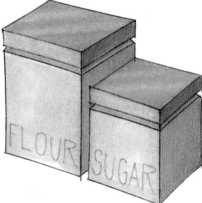

Periodically, check the sell-by dates and use by dates on the packages of food stored in your pantry. If things are past this date or if they look suspect in any way (dented cans, cracked jars, seeping contents, missing lids, and so on), throw them away!

how to

organize

your

pantry

* Take all of your food from the various spots where it's currently housed and put it onto your table. Throw away anything that is past its sell-by or use-by date, is stale, or looks suspect in any way. Donate anything that is still edible but unwanted to your local food pantry.

* Clean the shelves and walls of the pantry. Install new shelving (if needed), wire racks for additional storage solutions, and wall-mounted wire organizers. These items are available at your favorite retailer and at many supermarkets as well.

* Use canisters to store large bulk items such as flour, sugar, tea, and coffee. If these canisters do not have labels, label them. Don't forget to include the use-by date.

* Put spices together on a wall-mounted rack attached on the inside of the door or on a lazy Susan for easy access.

* When purchasing containers, choose square ones over round ones, as they fit more efficiently on shelves, resulting in better use of space.

* Always have backups of frequently used staples on hand, such as spaghetti, coffee, tea bags, mayonnaise, mustard, and so on.

* Keep a small notepad or chalkboard in your pantry to record when you use something up. Use this record to help create your shopping list, and avoid having to go back to the store because you forgot you were out of tuna!

What's the Dish?

The cabinets used to store your dishes, pots, pans, and small appliances should be organized by function and frequency of use. Put things used to prepare food in one cabinet, and things used to serve and eat food in another. Your fine china, seasonal serving pieces, and similar items should be stored in the upper recesses of your cabinets that are not within easy reach. To protect your grandma's good china or Aunt Minnie's turkey platter, either wrap the pieces individually in acid-free tissue to avoid chipping and scratching, or buy quilted dish-storage units at your favorite home-furnishings store or organizational shop. Dishes that you use every day should be stored within easy reach.

TIP OF THE TRADE: A safe and inexpensive way to store stacked dishes, to help prevent chipping and scratching, is to place a paper plate or small square of felt between each dish. If you don't have any paper plates or would rather not purchase felt, paper napkins or paper towels can also be used.

Pots and pans should be stored in the cabinets nearest your stove or oven. These can be stacked inside one another, with lids stored on a small rack that can be attached to the inside of the cabinet door. Also, if you're short on cabinet space, consider getting a pot rack, which is available in the housewares section of most major retailers. These range in style from countertop to wall- or ceiling-mounted versions. Decide which one is right for you on the basis of your personal needs and the amount of space you have for the rack. Specialty or infrequently used pots and pans such as pressure cookers, baking items, and seasonal cookery should be stored in hard-to-reach cabinets or less-used areas of your kitchen to allow more space for your everyday cookware.

Small appliances such as hand mixers, blenders, food processors, and the like should be stored where they can be accessed when you need them. Often, these appliances have many parts (and occasionally a detachable electrical cord) that should be stored with the appliance, to avoid loss or damage. A blender without its lid can turn your summer frozen-margarita party into a disaster.

MUSIC, FILM, VIDEO

Storing your CDs, DVDs, and VHS tapes (or maybe your record albums, 8-tracks, or even Betamax tapes) can be simplified by—just as with your clothes—editing and organizing them. Follow these simple steps to have the best media library in town!

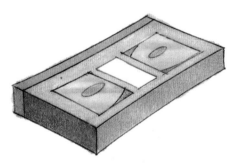

* Scour your home, car, office, and briefcase to gather all of your favorite CDs or videos. Throw out any that are scratched or damaged, and put the ones you don't want into a separate pile to donate to your favorite thrift shop or give away to your friends. Put the right discs or videos in the right packages. If any of the plastic packages are cracked, get new ones at your favorite music or video-rental store. Don't forget to label the package on the front and the spine.

* Separate into categories (for music: classical, pop, rock, show tunes, hip-hop, jazz, R&B; for videos/DVDs: comedies, romance, dramas, thrillers, classics, television). If you are über-organized, you may want to alphabetize by title or artist.

* Place items on a shelf, spine out for easy selection. If you don't have a media cabinet with a shelf, you may want to buy a carrier

or stand designed specifically to hold DVDs, CDs, or VHS tapes. Many people like to store their CDs or DVDs in large soft-sided albums with pages that have plastic pockets to hold the discs (without their cases). These albums can be separated by style of music or type of video and stored on a shelf, in a drawer, or in any other convenient spot in your home.

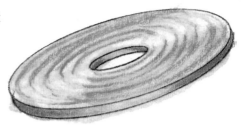

THE WINE CELLAR

The ultimate in attainable luxury is to have your own personal wine cellar. However, if you don't have the space for one, a nice wine rack, available from your favorite furniture or department store, or a shelf in your closet will suffice for short-term storage (six months or less).

To make your collection accessible and easily inventoried, keep types of wine together: Store reds with reds, white with whites. Never store wine in direct sunlight, as this will cause the wine to break down and lose its taste. Write the date that the wine was purchased on the label so that you know how long a bottle's been hanging around. Avoid storing wine near your stove or dishwasher, where pockets of high heat can affect it. Wine needs a cool, dark place for optimum storage. Also, store your wines low to the ground or in a cabinet away from overhead fluorescent lighting, which can also damage it, affecting its taste and shelf life. Avoid storing wine on top of your refrigerator; the proximity to the overhead lighting and the constant vibration can affect the flavor.

Many wines today come with screw caps and rubber corks, meaning that the wine can be stored standing up. However, many wines are still being produced with natural cork. These should be stored on their side to keep the wine inside the bottle in constant contact with the cork to maintain an airtight seal and protect the contents from oxygen and outside aromas. Never store bottles upside down, as the sediment may collect on the cork. And once you have opened a bottle of wine and have some left over, never return it to its original storage place. Recork it using the original end of the cork back in the bottle (if it has expanded, shave it down with a knife) or buy an inexpensive bottle stopper at your favorite liquor or grocery store (they usually cost less than $2) and place the opened bottle in the refrigerator. The bottles can stand upright because the seal has already been broken. Most white wines will last for three days in the refrigerator, while most reds will last for a day or two.

TIP OF THE TRADE: The optimum storage temperature is 45 degrees Fahrenheit for white wine and 55 degrees Fahrenheit for red wine.

EASY LIVING

Today our homes have to serve many purposes and provide flexibility to fit our hectic schedules. Everyone, from the single busy professional living in a small urban studio apartment to the surburban family living in a large, custom-designed home, needs their space to be functional and usable. Specialized areas such as wine cellars, home gymnasiums, dressing rooms/ custom closets, and others further streamline our lives, making each day easier and making our living space more adaptable to our lifestyles and more user-friendly than ever before. The ideas and designs created for the high-end market can be easily translated and transferred to anyone's living space. Is a custom-designed wine cellar out of the question financially? With your new found storage know-how, organize and store your favorite bottles in a corner of your apartment. Can't afford a custom-designed walk-in (the ultimate) closet? Use the ideas from this book to set up even the smallest reach-in so it works for you. Peruse those glossy shelter magazines, study brochures for custom-built homes, and read up on all the latest design and lifestyle trends, and then use them to improve your living space. In the process, you'll make your life better and more reflective of you and how you live it!

custom living spaces

In the high-end residential market, we are seeing ever-increasing specialization. It's not just the increasing size of the home but also the customization of the spaces to meet the needs of busy style-conscious clients. For instance, what once was a family room is often three to five separate rooms, each with its own set of requirements and areas of specialization. The media room, the gym, his-and-her offices, the kids' area—each has its own set of functional and aesthetic requirements. The same applies to the master suite and its surrounding spaces, such as his-and-her bathrooms and dressing areas. In talking about closet and organizational needs, it's not just about the clothes; it's about when you come rushing home, where do you put the mail? Your keys? Your cell phone? How can you find the right shirt and tie combination? How can you decide which shoes to wear? In the high-end market, it's absolutely about great design, but it's also about efficiency and organization for super busy people.

David Cohen, president
the I. Grace Company, Commissioned Private
Residences, Inc.

BOOK 'EM, DAN-O

Think of your bookshelves or bookcases as a closet without doors. Organizing your books and objects on your bookshelves can improve the overall look of your home's décor and make your personal library easy and fun to use. Follow these easy steps to create the ultimate look for your book collection.

* If you have a lot of well-worn and unsightly paperbacks in your collection, consider passing the ones you've already read on to a friend or donating them to a local book drive or thrift shop. The ones you'd like to keep can be placed spine up in a basket or bin stored next to your favorite chair to encourage reading, or in another spot within your home.

* Start by placing the larger books on the shelves first. Varying heights of objects on a flat surface excite the eye and make for more interesting viewing, so instead of placing the books in descending size order, why not try placing the larger books toward the center of the shelves and the smaller books toward the ends?

* If your books have dust jackets, keep them on them, as they might get lost if removed. (Collectible books lose a great deal of their value if their original dust jacket has been lost or thrown away.) However, if you prefer a more classic look where the leather binding shows, save your book jackets in a place where they can be retrieved and placed back on on the books if the need arises.

* Place some of the books on the shelf horizontally instead of

vertically. This arrangement allows for the horizontal books to hold up the vertical ones and provides a nice buildup (platform or stage) for a decorative object to enhance the bookshelf.

* Use decorative objects such as boxes, statues, souvenirs, memorabilia, and favorite collectibles interspersed with the books to add visual interest and appeal. Framed photographs, artwork, and small pieces of sculpture can also be used to break up the line of books on a shelf. Remember to keep the number to a minimum (you don't want to create a mass of clutter or wind up with a tableau reminiscent of a garage-sale display) and choose objects of varying heights and shapes for visual and decorative interest.

* You can place plants on the shelf to add a splash of color and life to your tableau. (Don't forget to put a dish or plate under the plant to avoid wetting the neighboring books when the plant is watered!)

* Placing a small lamp on a shelf to throw a pool of light further enhances the ambiance of your bookshelf and provides additional light to help you select a title.

There are so many areas of your home that we haven't even talked about—your refrigerator, your vanity, your garage, your desk. The possibilities are endless. But whichever cluttered, disheveled space it is, follow the principles of *Shop Your Closet* and let this book be your daily guide in your quest to attain the ultimate goal—organizational nirvana. Happy organizing!

RESOURCES

Alvin Valley
www.alvinvalley.com

Amrita Singh
www.amritasingh.com

Behnaz Sarafpour
www.behnazsarafpour.com

Carolina Herrera
www.carolinaherrera.com

Celerie Kemble
www.kembleinteriors.com

Christian Dior
www.christiandior.fr

Christian Loboutin
www.christianlouboutin.fr

Earnest Sewn
www.earnestsewn.com

Ferguson & Shamamian Architects
www.fergusonshamamian.com

Francesca Romana
www.francescaromana.com

House of Torn
www.houseoftorn.com

Hudson Jeans
www.hudsonjeans.com

Isaia
www.isaia.it

Kathryn Forest Design
www.kathrynforestdesign.com

Lara Hélène Bridal Atelier
www.larahelene.com

Michael Kors
www.michaelkors.com

Miguelina Gambaccini
www.miguelina.com

Milly
www.millyny.com

Noel Jeffrey
www.noeljeffrey.com

Peter Som
www.petersom.com

Roger Ferris + Partners
www.ferrisarch.com

Shoshanna
www.shoshanna.com

Starr Haymes
www.opusinteriors.com

Steve Gambrel
www.srgambrel.com

Theory
www.theory.com

Tibi
www.tibi.com

Tory Burch
www.toryburch.com

FASHION CONSULTANTS

Wendy Hirschberg Clurman
wendyhirschbergclurman
@gmail.com

FUR/CLOTHING STORAGE

Garde Robe
www.garderobeonline.com

ONLINE RETAILERS/ AUCTIONS

eBay
www.ebay.com

Net-A-Porter
www.net-a-porter.com

Portero
www.portero.com

Shopbop
www.shopbop.com

Vivre
www.vivre.com

NOT-FOR-PROFIT ORGANIZATIONS

Dress for Success
www.dressforsuccess.org

Goodwill
www.goodwill.org

Housing Works
www.housingworks.org

One World Running
http://oneworldrunning.blogspot.com

Salvation Army
www.salvationarmyusa.org

Society of St. Vincent de Paul
www.svdpusa.org

Vietnam Veterans of America
www.clothingdonations.org/service.htm

REAL ESTATE/ DEVELOPMENT

David Cohen, I. Grace Company
www.igrace.com

Michael Shvo NYC
www.shvo.com

John Rogers, Woolems, Inc.
jrogers@woolemsinc.com

Heather Woolems, Sotheby's Realty
heather.woolems@
sothebysrealty.com

J. Woolems, Woolems, Inc.
jwoolems@woolemsinc.com

RETAILERS

American Tourister
www.americantourister.com

Artbag Creations, Inc.
www.artbag.com

Barneys
www.barneys.com

Bergdorf Goodman
www.bergdorfgoodman.com

Calypso
www.calypso-celle.com

Container Store—Elfa Storage
www.containerstore.com

Flight 001
www.flight001.com

Ghurka
www.ghurka.com

Hold Everything
www.holdeverything.com

Home Depot
www.homedepot.com

Ina—consignment
www.inanyc.com

Kiehl's
www.kiehls.com

Lowe's
www.lowes.com

Neiman Marcus
www.neimanmarcus.com

Saks Fifth Avenue
www.saksfifthavenue.com

Samsonite
www.samsonite.com

T. Anthony Ltd.
www.tanthony.com

Tie Crafters
www.tiecrafters.com

Tumi
www.tumi.com

STYLISTS

Lauren Davis
laurenkdavis@mac.com

Tinsley Mortimer
mercermortimer@aol.com

Wardrobe-NYC, Neva Lindner
www.wardrobe-nyc.com

This is the inventory chart I fill out with my clients so they can get a handle on what's in their closet. Use it to catalogue your own wardrobe and don't be afraid to customize it to fit your individual needs and reflect your clothing inventory.

RESOURCES

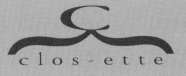

CLIENT INVENTORY ASSESSMENT

HERS		ITEM COUNT	LINEAR INCHES	QUALITY AND SIZE OF DRAWERS	NOTES
Hanging	Pants				
	Shirts				
	Jackets/blazers				
	Suits				
	Coats				
	Long dresses				
	Shorter dresses				
	Skirts				
	Other				
Folded	Bulky sweaters				
	Slim sweaters				
	T-shirts				
	Activewear/ workout clothes				
	Pants/jeans				
	Sleepwear				
Accessories	Underwear				
	Socks/stockings				
	Jewelry				
	Belts/gloves/etc.				
	Scarves/shawls				
	Bathing suits				
Shoes	Tall Boots				
	Low-mid boots				
	Flats				
Other Items					

HIS		ITEM COUNT	LINEAR INCHES	QUALITY AND SIZE OF DRAWERS	NOTES
Hanging	Pants				
	Shirts				
	Jackets/blazers				
	Suits				
	Coats				
	Other				
Folded	Bulky sweaters				
	Slim sweaters				
	T-shirts				
	Activewear/ workout clothes				
	Pants/jeans				
	Sleepwear				
	Bathing suits				
Accessories	Underwear				
	Socks/stockings				
	Belts/gloves/etc.				
	Briefcases/bags				
	Ties				
Shoes	Boots				
	Shoes				
Other Items					

INDEX